SpringerBriefs in Social Work

SpringerBriefs in Social Work and Social Change

AF800474

Series Editors

Rajendra Baikady, Department of Social Work
Central University of Kerala
Kasargod, Kerala, India

Jaroslaw Przeperski, Centre for Family Research
Nicolaus Copernicus University
Torun, Poland

S. M. Sajid, Department of Social Work
Jamia Millia Islamia
New Delhi, India

SpringerBriefs in Social Work and Social Change is a compact book series of authored and edited briefs on the state-of-the-art literature on social work and social change as well as globalization and social change, neoliberalism and social change, and societal response to social change, with special reference to social work education, research and practice.

The principal aim of the Series is to examine social change in a constantly changing world with new economic, political and social orders and how social work as a human service profession responds to these changes. Contributions in this Series go beyond accepting change as an inevitable force and reflect on our power in influencing, redirecting and contemplating social change. It is with this principal aim that we call upon academia, policy-makers, researchers and educators in social work, at all levels of their career stage, to explore the positive part of social change; i.e., what can we learn from social change while revisiting its negativity and impact.

Volumes published in this Series approach social change at different levels of society (whether local, regional, national, transnational, or at the macro, meso and micro levels). The Series identifies and defines the concept of social change within the social work context and its impact on human development at various national and international scopes.

Featuring compact volumes of 55 to 125 pages, *SpringerBriefs in Social Work and Social Change* is a comprehensive collection of high-quality literature on social change, with a primary focus on social work, contributed by educators, researchers, and practitioners across the globe. Both solicited and unsolicited manuscripts are considered for publication in this Series.

Muhammed Jabir • Anoop C. Choolayil

Social Work with Populations Vulnerable to Neglected Tropical Diseases

Evidence and Insights from India

Springer

Muhammed Jabir
Epidemiology and Operational Research
ICMR-Vector Control Research Centre
Puducherry, India

Anoop C. Choolayil
One Health
ICMR-Vector Control Research Centre
Puducherry, India

ISSN 2195-3104 ISSN 2195-3112 (electronic)
SpringerBriefs in Social Work
ISSN 2731-0760 ISSN 2731-0779
SpringerBriefs in Social Work and Social Change
ISBN 978-3-031-68996-3 ISBN 978-3-031-68997-0 (eBook)
https://doi.org/10.1007/978-3-031-68997-0

© The Editor(s) (if applicable) and The Author(s), under exclusive license to Springer Nature Switzerland AG 2024

This work is subject to copyright. All rights are solely and exclusively licensed by the Publisher, whether the whole or part of the material is concerned, specifically the rights of translation, reprinting, reuse of illustrations, recitation, broadcasting, reproduction on microfilms or in any other physical way, and transmission or information storage and retrieval, electronic adaptation, computer software, or by similar or dissimilar methodology now known or hereafter developed.
The use of general descriptive names, registered names, trademarks, service marks, etc. in this publication does not imply, even in the absence of a specific statement, that such names are exempt from the relevant protective laws and regulations and therefore free for general use.
The publisher, the authors and the editors are safe to assume that the advice and information in this book are believed to be true and accurate at the date of publication. Neither the publisher nor the authors or the editors give a warranty, expressed or implied, with respect to the material contained herein or for any errors or omissions that may have been made. The publisher remains neutral with regard to jurisdictional claims in published maps and institutional affiliations.

This Springer imprint is published by the registered company Springer Nature Switzerland AG
The registered company address is: Gewerbestrasse 11, 6330 Cham, Switzerland

If disposing of this product, please recycle the paper.

Foreword

The United Nations Sustainable Development Goal 3 (SDG 3) aims to achieve health and wellbeing for all by 2030. However, health services, health systems and healthcare facilities in most countries are becoming expensive despite advancements in science and technology, new innovations and paradigm shifts in medical systems. In the midst of growing inequality and disparity across nations and population groups, safeguarding minimum basic welfare, such as good health and wellbeing, is imperative to any country in its way towards development. Our global society experienced the worst public health challenge, namely COVID-19, which the World Health Organization declared a pandemic in March 2020. During the time of the pandemic, most countries in the world came to understand the shortcomings in their healthcare facilities and healthcare management. The COVID-19 pandemic also worsened the already existing global health inequality, in which countries in the Global South were experiencing the most difficult challenges due to their resource and leadership deficits. The pandemic provided an opportunity for policy makers and administrators to understand that the investment in public health and the wellbeing of people should not go unnoticed.

This book, written by Muhammed Jabir and Anoop C. Choolayil, brings fresh discussion on aspects related to social work practices with populations vulnerable to neglected tropical diseases (NTDs). It consists of five chapters that outline the current situation of NTDs in India. The authors open the discussion with a global overview of NTDs, the challenges in addressing NTDs and the role of social work in controlling and eliminating NTDs. The discussion in Chap. 2 provides more detail related to India and offers an understanding to readers on the social dimensions of health and illness. Furthermore, the authors also discuss health equality and the impact of heath inequality in Indian society, with special reference to populations vulnerable to NTDs. While NTDs are common in developing and less developed countries, their impact on vulnerable population groups in India cannot be neglected. With limited health facilities and poor access to clean water and basic sanitation, housing and nutrition for most vulnerable population groups, addressing the impact of NTDs on the overall wellbeing of these groups in India is timely and important.

As the authors highlight in their book, social work intervention with populations vulnerable to NTDs is important for achieving a just and equal society where no one is left behind. Furthermore, social justice and human dignity are the core principles on which the social work profession is established and practised across the globe. Social workers, as human service professionals, strive to ensure access to equal, meaningful and participatory opportunities for all sections of society. Social work provides a range of services in both the physical and mental health areas. However, in our contemporary society, the role of social work is not well recognized and respected in several countries. In India, even 87 years after its birth, social work is unable to achieve professional status; nevertheless, through various forms, the profession is profoundly impacting millions of people who are marginalized and vulnerable in contemporary India.

Throughout this book, authors Muhammed Jabir and Anoop C. Choolayil highlighted the importance of developing innovative and impactful social work interventions and practices to address NTDs. Social workers need to understand the social conditions and economic situations that increase people's vulnerability in terms of health and wellbeing. Furthermore, their ability to understand social dimensions such as poverty, cultural practices, and social identity among different communities in India significantly influences their intervention with these population groups. Social workers play a pivotal role in strengthening societies through social work interventions and participatory social development. To address growing health and wellbeing concerns, India needs to strengthen its human services profession, such as social workers and allied health professionals.

In conclusion, I remind readers that social work as a human service profession can bring desirable and impactful change to our society when we believe in the power of human dignity, human worth and human rights. Accordingly, modern social work educational programmes and training should focus on developing professionally trained and ethically competent workforces to serve the neediest population groups of our society.

Rajendra Baikady, PhD, FRSA

Central University of Kerala
Kasargod, Kerala, India
University of Johannesburg
Johannesburg, South Africa
York University
Toronto, ON, Canada
24 June 2024

Contents

About the Authors

Muhammed Jabir is a Social Scientist (Scientist-B) in the Department of Epidemiology and Operational Research at the Indian Council of Medical Research - Vector Control Research Centre, Puducherry, India. He holds a PhD in social work from the Delhi School of Social Work, University of Delhi. Before joining ICMR, he was teaching at the Madras School of Social Work, Chennai. His research primarily focuses on exploring the social and behavioural determinants of health, with a particular interest in how community engagement and social science approaches can play an essential role in preventing and controlling vector-borne diseases.

Anoop C. Choolayil is a Social Scientist (Scientist-B) at the Vector Control Research Centre of the Indian Council of Medical Research (ICMR-VCRC), Puducherry, India. He holds a PhD in Social Work from the Central University of Kerala and postgraduate degrees in Social Work and Psychology. As a dedicated public health professional trained in health social work, he works towards advancing health equity through targeted interventions among communities endemic to Neglected Tropical Diseases, particularly Vector-borne Diseases. He is actively implementing multiple research projects that work towards improving the health prospects of marginalised communities. His research interests include health equity, health policy, human rights and gerontology.

Chapter 1
Neglected Tropical Diseases: A Brief Introduction to the Global Scenario

1.1 Introduction

Ever since the Universal Declaration of Human Rights, health has increasingly been recognised as a human right, and health equity has been considered the means to achieve this right. However, the concept of health equity originated and was a major subject matter in social medicine much before the UDHR was in place. The concept of health equity can be traced back to the mid-nineteenth century to the works of Rudolf Virchow, Friedrich Engels and Andrija Stampar, who emphasised the role of social inequalities in perpetuating health inequity (Fee & Gonzalez, 2017). The concept of health equity started gaining traction after the World Health Organization's Constitution emphasised that the accessibility to the highest standards of health should be available to all without discrimination (WHO, 1946) and 2 years later, in 1948, enshrined health as a human right in the Universal Declaration of Human Rights (Meltsner, 1966; Yao et al., 2019). However, the studies on health equity started accelerating only after the 1990s. Currently, though the terms 'health disparity', 'health inequality' and 'health inequity' are interchangeably used, the term 'health inequity' is considered most appropriate as it captures the preventable and unnecessary disparities in health that can be prevented (Arcaya et al., 2015). Health inequity would, thus, mean systematic differences that people across different social domains experience in the domain of health (Hill, 2016), and equity in healthcare refers to the equality in access, utilisation and quality of care available for all (Yao et al., 2019). Health equity is considered the foundational idea in ensuring health as a human right for all. The concept is important given the fact that globally, a wide array of diseases are attributed to being induced by poor living conditions and other social determinants.

Neglected tropical diseases (NTDs) involve a case of health inequity associated with the social determinants of health. NTDs are facilitated by poor accessibility to essential resources like clean water and proper housing. Health inequities and

© The Author(s), under exclusive license to Springer Nature Switzerland AG 2024
M. Jabir, A. C. Choolayil, *Social Work with Populations Vulnerable to Neglected Tropical Diseases*, SpringerBriefs in Social Work,
https://doi.org/10.1007/978-3-031-68997-0_1

disparities emerging from such disparities create poor health outcomes for billions of people globally. NTDs are a diverse group of diseases that are prevalent in tropical areas, affecting more than a billion people. NTDs are typical in impoverished settings where people lack resources and are entangled in poverty. Mostly limited to the tropics, NTDs represent intersecting poverty and other disadvantages. The term 'neglected' symbolises the historical disparities in global health priorities that prioritised a few infectious diseases like HIV/AIDS and tuberculosis but gave little to no attention to the cluster of diseases that are now termed NTDS (Hotez et al., 2020; Hotez, 2021). NTDs have often languished in the shadows, and the diseases in the NTD spectrum disproportionately impact populations with limited access to healthcare, sanitation and education, perpetuating a cycle of poverty and ill health. The idea of neglected tropical diseases was first introduced after the adoption of the Millennium Development Goals in the early 2000s, which particularly emphasised the need for the elimination of diseases like HIV/AIDS and tuberculosis but neglected several other tropical diseases with substantial global prevalence. In response to this, a set of thirteen "neglected" infectious diseases were collectively categorised under the umbrella of NTDs (Hotez & Lo, 2020; Molyneux et al., 2005). NTDs span a diverse range of diseases with unique aetiologies, modes of transmission and clinical manifestations. Originally encompassing thirteen diseases, the scope of NTDs has been fluctuating, with WHO's list of twenty NTDs being the one with the greater consensus. The list of NTDs, according to the World Health Organization, includes Buruli ulcer, Chagas disease, dengue and chikungunya, dracunculiasis (Guinea-worm disease), echinococcosis, foodborne trematodiases, human African trypanosomiasis (sleeping sickness), leishmaniasis, leprosy (Hansen's disease), lymphatic filariasis, mycetoma, chromoblastomycosis and other deep mycoses, onchocerciasis (river blindness), podoconiosis, rabies, scabies and other ectoparasitoses, schistosomiasis, soil-transmitted helminthiases, snakebite envenoming, taeniasis/cysticercosis, trachoma and yaws and other endemic treponematoses (WHO, 2023). The World Health Organization (WHO) has categorised neglected tropical diseases (NTDs) into two distinct groups: Preventive Chemotherapy and Transmission Control (PCT) NTDs, and Innovative and Intensified Disease Management (IDM) NTDs, for the purpose of control and elimination programmes. The primary approach for controlling PCT diseases, including lymphatic filariasis, onchocerciasis, schistosomiasis and soil-transmitted helminthiasis, involves mass drug administration (MDA). IDM NTDs involve those that currently lack suitable tools for large-scale implementation, such as Buruli ulcer, Chagas disease, human African trypanosomiasis and leishmaniasis (Mitra & Mawson, 2017). These NTDs, their mode of transmission and causative organisms are listed in Table 1.1.

NTDs are distinctively distributed geographically, with the burden of these diseases primarily affecting the tropical and subtropical regions around the world (Hotez et al., 2020; Hotez, 2014). The geographical distribution of the diseases is shaped by the intersection of specific environmental conditions, poverty and inadequate healthcare infrastructure. Sub-Saharan Africa is burdened with NTDs, including malaria, schistosomiasis, lymphatic filariasis and onchocerciasis. The

Table 1.1 Major NTDs listed by the World Health Organization

Sl. No.	NTDs	Transmission/risk factors	Pathogen
1.	Buruli ulcer	Unknown	Bacteria: *Mycobacterium ulcerans*
2.	Chagas disease	Vector: Triatomine bugs	Parasite: *Trypanosoma cruzi*
3.	Dengue fever	Vector: *Aedes* mosquitoes (*Aedes aegypti* and *Aedes albopictus*)	Virus (Flavivirus): Dengue virus
	Chikungunya	Vector: *Aedes* mosquitoes (*Aedes aegypti* and *Aedes albopictus*)	Virus (Flavivirus): Chikungunya virus
4.	Dracunculiasis	Contaminated water	Parasite: *Dracunculus medinensis* or Guinea-worm
5.	Echinococcosis Cystic echinococcosis Alveolar echinococcosis	Faeces of dogs, foxes and other carnivores	Parasite: Cystic echinococcosis: *Echinococcus granulosus* Alveolar echinococcosis: *Echinococcus multilocularis*
6.	Food-borne trematodiases	Contaminated food (raw fish, crustaceans or vegetables)	Parasites: *Clonorchis, Opisthorchis, Fasciola* and *Paragonimus*
7.	Human African trypanosomiasis	Vector: Tsetse flies (*Glossina spp.*) (African)	Parasite: *Trypanosoma brucei* (African)
8.	Leishmaniasis	Vector: Phlebotomine sandflies (*Phlebotomine spp.*)	Parasite: Various *Leishmania* species *L. donovani* complex (3 species) *L. mexicana* complex (3 main species) *L. tropica*; *L. major*; *L. aethiopica*; and the subgenus *Viannia* with 4 main species
9.	Leprosy	Droplets from the nose and mouth through prolonged contact with untreated cases	Bacteria: *Mycobacterium leprae*
10.	Lymphatic filariasis	Vector (mosquitoes): *Culex spp., Anopheles spp., Mansonia spp., Aedes spp.*	Parasite: *Wuchereria bancrofti, Brugia malayi, Brugia timori*
11.	Mycetoma, chromoblastomycosis and other deep mycoses	Traumatic inoculation of certain fungi or bacteria into the subcutaneous tissue	Mycetoma: bacteria (actinomycetoma) or fungi (eumycetoma) Chromoblastomycosis: pigmented fungi, most commonly *Fonsecaea pedrosoi, Fonsecaea monophora* and *Cladophialophora carrionii* Sporotrichosis: fungus *Sporothrix*
12.	Onchocerciasis (River Blindness)	Vector: Blackflies (*Simulium spp.*)	Parasite: *Onchocerca volvulus*

(continued)

Table 1.1 (continued)

Sl. No.	NTDs	Transmission/risk factors	Pathogen
13.	Cancrum oris or gangrenous stomatitis (noma)	Poor oral hygiene, malnutrition and weakened immune system	Non-specific polymicrobial organisms associated with social determinants
14.	Rabies	Zoonotic: exposure to rabid domestic and wild animals via contact with saliva usually through bites, scratches or direct contact with mucosa	Virus: *Lyssavirus Rabies*
	Scabies and other ectoparasitoses	Infection with a microscopic mite through close contact with the skin	Parasite: *Sarcoptes scabiei var hominis*
15.	Schistosomiasis	Vector: Snails	Schistosoma species (*S. mansoni, S. haematobium, S. japonicum, S. intercalatum, S. mekongi*)
16.	Soil-transmitted helminthiases	Transmitted by eggs present in human faeces, which contaminate the soil in areas where sanitation is poor	parasitic worms: *Ascaris lumbricoides, Trichuris trichiura, Necator americanus* and *Ancylostoma duodenale*
17.	Snakebite envenoming	Snakebite	–
18.	Taeniasis/cysticercosis	Poor hygiene (via the faecal-oral route) or ingesting contaminated food or water	Parasitic worms: *Taenia solium, Taenia saginata and Taenia asiatica*
19.	Trachoma	Personal contact (via hands, clothes, bedding or hard surfaces) and by flies that have been in contact with discharge from the eyes or nose of an infected person	Bacterium: *Chlamydia trachomatis*
20.	Yaws	Person to person	Bacterium: *Treponema pallidum* subspecies *pertenue*

Source: WHO (n.d.) Neglected tropical diseases

prevalence estimates suggest that at least half a billion of the Sub-Saharan population is burdened by NTDs (George et al., 2023). Southeast Asia, with its warm and humid climate, is also home to multiple NTDs, including dengue, lymphatic filariasis and soil-transmitted helminthiasis. All 11 countries in the Southeast Asia Region (SEAR) are affected by NTDs, and the region bears 54 per cent of the global burden of NTDs, with 15 of the 20 NTDs present in the region (Yajima et al., 2023). Latin America and the Caribbean region have cases of soil-transmitted helminth infection and Chagas disease as the most prevalent NTDs, followed by diseases like dengue, leishmaniasis and lymphatic filariasis (Hotez et al., 2008). The West Pacific region has a burden of 15 NTDs endemic to 28 countries in the Western Pacific region (WHO, 2020). Some of the major diseases burdening the region include filariasis, soil-transmitted helminthiasis and dengue. The Middle East and North Africa (MENA) region is marked by high endemicity but patchily distribution of NTDs among the 20 countries of the MENA region. Some of the major diseases reported in the region are soil-transmitted nematode infections, filarial infections, schistosomiasis, etc. (Hotez et al., 2012). In the South Asia region, NTDs constitute a significant part of the overall disease burden, significantly affecting the economic progress of the South Asian countries (Singh, 2017). Nearly one billion South Asians living in poverty suffer from NTDs, accounting for one-quarter of the soil-transmitted helminth infections and at least half of the lymphatic filariasis, visceral leishmaniasis and leprosy burden globally (Lobo et al., 2011).

The prevalence of NTDs is associated with social determinants of health, such as poverty, level of education and limited access to clean water and sanitation. NTDs are common in conditions where environmental factors, like the presence of vectors, reservoirs and hosts, confluence with socioeconomic factors like poverty and resource scarcity that limit the ability of a community to protect itself (Hotez, 2021; Garchitorena et al., 2017). One of the defining features of NTDs is the limited arsenal of effective treatments. For many of the NTDs, the current treatments are not adequate, and for some, there are few or no treatments available (De Rycker et al., 2018). One of the major reasons for the limited treatment options is the perceived low profitability among pharma companies and, hence, limited research and development in the domain (Jung et al., 2020). Consequently, many affected populations face challenges in accessing even basic treatments. Table 1.1 lists the major NTDs recognised by the WHO (n.d.) along with the transmission mode or risk factor along with the pathogens inducing them.

1.2 Impact of NTDs on Affected Populations

Since NTDs are a cluster of diverse diseases, their impact cannot be comprehensively summarised in uniform terms. However, the adverse outcomes these diseases create for the affected population are evident beyond debate. In economic terms, NTDs pose a significant financial burden on developing economies, accounting for huge losses in revenue every year by disrupting productivity in agricultural and industrial labour, hindering the earning capacity of individuals who are already living in poverty and surviving on less than two dollars a day (Mitra & Mawson, 2017). Since most NTDs lead to disabilities, they contribute to over 57 million Disability Adjusted Life Years (DALYs) (Ochola et al., 2021; Herricks et al., 2017; Hotez, 2009). However, DALYs do not capture all the political and socioeconomic consequences of NTDs (Ochola et al., 2021). In terms of adverse social outcomes, NTDs cast a long and often devastating shadow on the communities they afflict, perpetuating a cycle of poverty and ill health. The impact of NTDs is multifaceted, affecting individuals, families and entire populations and their physical, social, economic and psychological well-being. Some of the adverse impacts NTDs have on the affected populations are discussed below.

Morbidity and Disability: Many NTDs are notorious for causing chronic and debilitating conditions that result in long-term morbidity and disability. For instance, individuals affected by lymphatic filariasis may suffer from elephantiasis (severe swelling of limbs) and/or hydrocele (severe swelling of the scrotum), which can significantly impair mobility and overall quality of life (WHO, 2023). Trachoma infection can lead to corneal ulceration and can result in blindness (Kuper, 2019). NTDs lead to disabilities and add up to 57 million disability adjusted life years (DALYs) globally (Ochola et al., 2021; Herricks et al., 2017). Most NTDs result in disfiguring and disabling conditions that can result in permanent disability to the affected. Most intervention strategies target preventing transmission and ignore severe morbidities like lymphedema, disfigurement and blindness. Elimination targets should essentially address morbidity and help the population already affected by the NTDs (Deribe, 2015). Psycho-social interventions and Morbidity Management and Disability Prevention (MMDP) can be pivotal in this regard.

(a) *Economic Burden and Poor Productivity*: The chronic nature of NTDs adversely impacts the productivity of affected individuals. In the global context, particularly in the global south, NTDs result in significant financial losses accounting for billions of dollars to developing economies, mostly devastating the lives of individuals who are already living below the poverty line (Ochola et al., 2021). The disabilities like lymphedema and blindness caused by NTDs can significantly compromise functional capacity, leading to diminished productivity among affected individuals. Such disabling conditions can render individuals unable to participate in activities crucial to their livelihoods, such as farming or skilled labour. This loss of productivity extends to families and communities, exacerbating the economic burden on already marginalised populations.

(b) *Maternal and Child Health and Well-Being*: NTDs often have significant implications for reproductive health. Maternal and child health can sometimes be affected by NTDs to a great extent. Not all NTDs affecting the mother can pose significant threats to the child, but in cases like Chagas disease, the chances of congenital transmission exist (Kemmerling et al., 2019). Similarly, certain maternal hookworm infections are associated with adverse outcomes in pregnancy, contributing to maternal and child morbidity (Ness et al., 2020). Certain chronic infections, like intestinal helminthiasis, can lead to malnutrition and anaemia, hindering the physical and cognitive development of affected children (Degarege et al., 2022). Furthermore, the stigma associated with visible signs of certain NTDs, like skin lesions or deformities, can lead to social isolation and compromise a child's educational opportunities. Hence, children bear a disproportionate burden of several NTDs, impacting their growth, cognitive development and overall well-being.

(c) *Stigmatisation, Social Exclusion and Mental Health*: Many NTDS result in visible manifestations, sometimes disfiguring ones like skin lesions or blindness, which in turn can affect the mental health of the affected as these physical impairments not only limit functional capacity but also contribute to social stigma and discrimination. . Individuals with these visible signs may face discrimination, impacting their social relationships, marriage prospects and community integration. Stigmatisation contributes to the psychological burden of NTDs, exacerbating the mental health challenges faced by affected individuals. Depression, anxiety and feelings of hopelessness are not uncommon among those battling the physical and social ramifications of these diseases. The psychological burden extends to families and communities, compounding the overall impact on mental well-being.

(d) *Community Well-Being*: The collective impact of NTDs in endemic areas goes beyond individual suffering and impacts the overall well-being of communities that are affected. The economic productivity of affected populations is compromised, hindering community development. The burden on healthcare systems and limited resources directed toward NTD control further strain the resilience of communities grappling with these diseases. The overall health outcomes, productivity and well-being of communities can be adversely affected by NTDs. In fact, the communities that are affected by NTDs predominantly consist of impoverished populations lacking significant political influence to shape control initiatives (Ochola et al., 2022). Such communities are entrenched in a vicious cycle of poverty and ill health due to NTDs.

The impact of NTDs extends far beyond the physiological effects on individuals. It permeates through families and communities, shaping the socioeconomic fabric and perpetuating cycles of poverty and ill health. Addressing the multifaceted impact of NTDs requires holistic strategies that not only target the diseases themselves but also consider the broader determinants of health and well-being in affected populations. This necessitates interventions that address the social nature of the NTDs. Essentially, eliminating NTDs involves eliminating the adverse social determinants that pave way to increased vulnerability among the disadvantaged sections of society.

1.3 Neglected Tropical Diseases and the Role of Social Determinants

As discussed in previous sections, NTDs constitute one of the visible domains of global health disparities, reflecting a broader issue of inequitable distribution of resources and attention. The burden of NTDs results in individual suffering and perpetuates adverse outcomes for communities at large. Addressing neglected tropical diseases necessitates a comprehensive, interdisciplinary approach that goes beyond traditional disease-specific frameworks. Effective control strategies must consider environmental, social, and economic factors to break the transmission cycle and alleviate the burden on affected communities. Multiple social pathways, including illiteracy, malnutrition, poor living conditions and unemployment, are associated with getting infected with NTDs (Bishwajit et al., 2014). Some of the key social determinants associated with NTDs are discussed in the following section.

(a) *Socioeconomic Position (SEP)*: Perhaps the most important social determinant in terms of NTDs would be poor socioeconomic conditions. Poverty and poor health conditions have been found to be intertwined in such a manner that poverty induces poor health outcomes among vulnerable communities, and these poor health outcomes significantly deter the capability of the affected individuals and communities to prosper economically (Wagstaff, 2002). This is particularly true for NTDs where SEP and NTD infection are entangled, where SEP increases the odds of NTD infection and NTD infection, in turn, adversely affects SEP through income loss due to illness and associated costs (Houweling et al., 2016). SEP can serve as a causal factor in NTD infection through immediate determinants like hygiene practices, access to clean water and sanitation facilities, exposure to infection in occupational settings, etc., or through certain cofounding determinants like age and sex (Houweling et al., 2016). In either case, SEP serves as a critical determinant that makes people vulnerable to NTDs. This not only makes individuals vulnerable to NTDs but also affects the health services availed post-infection. Factors like poverty, geographical location, etc., can limit the treatment opportunities for people affected by NTDs. Socioeconomic position, in the case of NTDs, is not restricted to the individual level alone but extends to the community level as well. Groups of people belonging to certain sections of societies that are historically deprived of economic and social resources due to structural inequalities and intersecting disadvantages are often found to be affected by NTDs in many developing countries. The relationship between NTDs and poor SEP is not linear but cyclical, where suboptimal SEP induces vulnerability to NTDs and NTDs induce poor SEPs.
(b) *Behavioural Factors*: Cultural factors and behavioural traits entangle with SEP in the case of NTD infections. Behavioural elements contribute to contracting NTDs, and modification of certain behaviours can be helpful in preventing the infection and spread of NTDs. Sometimes, SEP indirectly leads to adverse behaviours like poor hygiene practices that favour the contraction and spread of NTDs. Water, sanitation and hygiene (WASH) are critical factors to human health, particularly in the case of NTDs. Healthy WASH practices reduce the risk of exposure to most disease vectors and are recognised as a major element in preventing NTDs (World Health Organization, 2015). Improved access to WASH infrastructure, however, does not necessarily ensure the prevention of NTDs; rather, infrastructural modification paired with WASH behavioural change can induce effective change (Parke et al., 2022). Similarly, preventive practices like avoiding contact with disease vectors also fall under the purview of behavioural factors that are associated with NTDs. Behavioural modifications that target to incorporate vector avoidance among people are hence a priority of most prevention programmes.

(c) *Environmental Factors*: The role of environmental characteristics in spreading NTDs is well recorded. The seasonality of many NTDs indicates the role of climatic and environmental factors in the propagation of NTDs. For instance, dengue infections are associated with rainfall and temperature to a great extent, complemented by infrastructural factors facilitating optimal breeding sites for dengue vectors (Raheel et al., 2011). Vector habitats are a key environmental factor associated with NTDs. While certain factors like vegetation, temperature, geographical features, etc., are unavoidable environmental characteristics facilitating NTDs, factors like stagnant water, climate change, etc., are human-made factors that contribute to adverse environmental characteristics facilitating NTDs. This is particularly true in the case of climate change, which is the most important human-induced environmental factor leading to NTDs, as most NTDs are caused by pathogens that are responsive to environmental conditions. Hence, the distribution patterns of most NTDs are influenced by climate change (Booth, 2018). Climate change will be one of the largest deciding factors in terms of NTDs in the upcoming decades.

(d) *Administrative and Policy Factors*: NTDs are, to a great extent, associated with intersecting structural deficits and disadvantages and hence require solid administrative and policy measures to achieve comprehensive control and elimination. The role of political action is widely acknowledged in the elimination of NTDs worldwide. The success of the current efforts to tackle NTDs owes to the mobilisation of the global health community by political leaders (Pastrana et al., 2020). Since NTDs are prevalent among marginalised communities that are often deprived of resources to modify their SEP or environmental conditions, the relevance of policy and administrative factors becomes relevant. The control of NTDs will essentially be more effective in societies that are governed by the ideology of a welfare state than in a state where the lowest strata of society are not paid enough attention. This happens due to the impact of policy decisions and resource allocation for the cause of NTD prevention and elimination by the state and its effective implementation through administrative channels.

The scope of the social nature of NTDs expands far beyond the factors explained in this section. Often, it is the intersection of multiple social determinants that can shape how NTDs affect and spread among communities. The very social nature of NTDs demands solutions that are social as well. While the mass drug administration (MDA) is considered an effective means to tackle most NTDs, interventions that are social in nature, leading to changes in the structural and individual disadvantages of affected individuals and communities, are quintessential in ensuring effective control and elimination of NTDs.

1.4 Challenges in the Control and Prevention of NTDs

While many diseases that troubled humanity have been addressed and tackled effectively through interventions like vaccinations and preventive mechanisms, NTDs have persisted over the years due to the complex nature of factors associated with their causation, transmission and sustenance. While some of the aspects are biological, some are social, indicating entangled social and biological determinants that make people vulnerable. Some of the key challenges associated with NTD control and prevention are discussed in the following section.

(a) *Vector Biology, Behaviour and Ecology*: The causative pathogens of many NTDs have intricate life cycles involving vectors such as mosquitoes, flies or other organisms. This complex cycle and dependence of the pathogen on vectors and intermediate hosts complicate the efforts of designing and implementing prevention strategies. Also, vector behaviour, including feeding habits, biting preferences and resting sites, pose challenges to the prevention of NTDs. For instance, *Aedes* mosquitoes are day-biting and hence using bed nets will not be an effective preventive measure. Hence, understanding the ecological niche and vector behaviour is a critical but extensive component in the prevention of NTDs. Likewise, understanding vector competence is also a critical component in managing NTDs effectively. Vector competence refers to the ability of a vector to acquire, sustain and transmit a pathogen, and understanding this will help control vectors more effectively. Understanding reservoirs of pathogens is another challenge in managing NTDs. Reservoirs maintain the pathogen in the environment, thereby providing a persistent source of reinfection, which makes eradication challenging (Peterson et al., 2020). Another critical concern associated with vector biology is insecticide resistance. Continued use of insecticides has made many vectors of NTDs resistant to traditional insecticides, posing a significant challenge to traditional control methods. Human actions leading to climate change are also constantly altering how vectors of many NTDs breed and expand to new ecological niches. These factors make NTD prevention and control a challenging task.

(b) *Healthcare Service and Infrastructure Limitations*: Globally, the healthcare infrastructure and resource distribution are often inadequate in addressing the burden of NTDs. In fact, NTDs like malaria and leishmaniasis are sometimes even facilitated by the breakdown of vector control programmes and health infrastructure (Chris et al., 2011). Besides, extensive surveillance and diagnosis mechanisms are essential in controlling NTDs due to the diverse nature and complex lifecycle of the pathogens, which is resource-intensive. Most countries affected by NTDs are developing and lack the resources to address the issue comprehensively (Ackley et al., 2021). In addition, NTDs and the efficacy of health services are linked (Marchal et al., 2011). In many cases, the healthcare system is overburdened and lacks resources to address the healthcare demand raised by the large influx created by the outbreak of certain NTDs like dengue. Hence, improving the healthcare infrastructure is essential to control NTDs, which needs intersectoral actions from multiple stakeholders. The method relied on for the control and elimination of many NTDs is preventive chemotherapy or mass drug administration (MDA), which are public health strategies involving the systematic administration of drugs to entire populations. However, despite its efficacy, MDAs sometimes fail to achieve the intended targets due to poor community compliance due to reasons like poor knowledge, fear of adverse effects, distrust in government programmes, etc. (Manyeh et al., 2020). Also, factors like limited vaccines, poor physical infrastructure, lack of manpower, etc., adversely affect global efforts to control NTDs. In addition, there are factors like the emergence of drug-resistant pathogens and limited pharmaceutical industry engagement that deter the goal of NTD elimination and prevention.

(c) *Complex Socioeconomic Determinants*: As discussed in the previous sections, NTDs and social determinants are entangled. Social determinants make people vulnerable to NTDs, and NTDs often worsen the socio-economic conditions of the affected. This cycle of entanglement makes NTDs difficult to tackle. This necessitates the modification of social determinants along with preventive chemotherapy. Since such modifications often require large-scale efforts at the infrastructural and societal levels, the state mechanisms often lag behind the required resources. Another challenge associated with socioeconomic development for the cause of NTD control and prevention is gaining political commitments (Yajima et al., 2023). However, gaining political commitment and allocation of funds is just the starting point; a complex set of socioeconomic determinants, including traditional practices of the target community, behavioural traits, occupational factors of individuals, etc., significantly influences the success of the implementation of most programmes. Hence, control and elimination of NTDs essentially involve socioeconomic challenges that need to be addressed at the policy and programme levels. Social and behavioural interventions by trained professionals become critical in this aspect. Methods like behaviour change communication (BCC) and social and behaviour change communication (SBCC) are helpful in bringing about changes at individual and community levels. However, larger structural changes require political commitments, policy modifications, adequate funding and effective implementation.

The prevention and control of neglected tropical diseases is a complex process due to the intricate relationships between pathogens, vectors and human hosts. Research into vector genetics, host-pathogen interactions, and innovative control strategies is essential for developing sustainable and effective interventions. However, the social determinants of NTDs are equally important and need attention to develop comprehensive strategies. Addressing the socio-economic determinants of NTDs and investing in healthcare infrastructure are crucial for achieving long-term success in NTD prevention efforts.

1.5 Global Efforts in Combating Neglected Tropical Diseases

Addressing NTDs requires a concerted global effort involving diverse stakeholders, including governments, international organisations, non-governmental organisations (NGOs), academia and the private sector. Global collaboration and partnerships are fundamental in mobilising resources, sharing knowledge and implementing effective strategies to control, eliminate and eventually eradicate NTDs. Some of the key efforts on the global stage to address NTDs are listed below:

(a) *WHO's NTD Roadmap*: The WHO introduced a roadmap to control and eliminate NTDs by introducing global and regional targets for 2020 (World Health Organization, 2012). The roadmap suggested five major interventions to overcome NTDs, viz., preventive chemotherapy, intensified case-detection and case management, vector and intermediate host control, veterinary public health and provision for safe water, sanitation and hygiene. The NTD roadmap was a major landmark as there was increased attention to NTDs on the global stage, and targeted actions were initiated globally. WHO proposed a new NTD roadmap in 2021 in order to attain Sustainable Development Goal (SDG) targets regarding NTDs. The attention of the new roadmap designed for 2021–2030 aims at increasing accountability for outcomes through impact indicators, transitioning from disease-specific initiatives to integrated programmes and facilitating programme ownership by respective countries (Warusavithana et al., 2022). The aim of the new roadmap was to identify critical gaps since 2010 and the actions required to achieve the 2030 targets effectively (World Health Organization, 2020). The NTD roadmap by the WHO is the benchmark when it comes to NTD control and elimination. The strategies adopted by member nations and other organisations rely on the NTD roadmap to set the targets and implement the interventions.

(b) *The London Declaration on Neglected Tropical Diseases*: Inspired by the WHO roadmap for NTDs, a global collaborative programme was launched by a group of pharmaceutical companies, certain philanthropic organisations, NGOs and affected countries. The objective was to establish networks and initiate collaborations to eradicate, eliminate or control NTDs. The pharmaceutical companies involved in the collaboration have steadily been donating medicines for the cause, and the philanthropic organisations have been allocating financial assistance to stakeholders involved. With the resources allocated by partnerships, the efforts to control NTDs are gaining momentum with a significant reduction in global burden.

(c) *Research Networks and Philanthropic Initiatives*: Multiple research collaborations have come into effect as a result of the World Health Organization's efforts to streamline the efforts to tackle NTDs. Initiatives like the Drugs for Neglected Diseases initiative (DNDi) and the Global Network for Neglected Tropical Diseases bring together researchers, institutions and pharmaceutical companies to drive drug discovery and development. Besides such research networks, multiple philanthropic organisations have committed significant funding to research, drug development and implementation programs targeting NTDs. These efforts have helped in tackling NTDs to a great extent at the global level.

There are multiple large-scale efforts globally that seek to address the question of controlling NTDs, which are contributing enormously to the cause of improving the lives of millions of people. In addition to such global initiatives, there are efforts at the grassroots levels, including non-governmental organisations (NGOs), civil society engagement, intersectoral collaborations and public-private partnerships that contribute to the cause of NTD elimination and control. The complex nature of NTDs requires coordinated efforts at the global and local levels, fostering partnerships that leverage diverse expertise and resources. With such efforts working towards combating NTDs, the cause of control and elimination shall be streamlined.

1.6 NTD Programmes and the Emerging Role of Social Work

One of the key challenges of NTD programmes is sustainability, i.e. the continued functioning of an NTD programme well beyond the period it is funded by an external agency (Madon et al., 2018). One of the most difficult tasks associated with NTD programmes is the fact that many programmes are not sustainable beyond the stipulated programme duration. Involving the community as a primary stakeholder in NTD implementation can help attain the goals of NTD programmes more effectively and sustain the programme. This can be addressed only by ensuring community participation and ownership in the NTD programme. However, community engagement and participation are difficult to attain due to multiple factors, including distrust in the health system, poor capacity of the frontline healthcare workforce, etc. (Madon et al., 2018). The poor community engagement in NTD programmes is often reflected in non-compliance and poor adherence to MDA programmes, which would otherwise successfully eliminate some of the NTDs (Halim et al., 2022). Ensuring community engagement in NTD programmes essentially involves social mobilisation efforts that are grounded in the social science disciplines.

Social work, as a discipline, has its origins in helping individuals attain health-related services and social workers have been working on social determinants of health, adding to the efforts of health equity and universal health coverage (Ruth & Marshall, 2017). NTD programmes often involve modification of social determinants of health (SDOH), and social work interventions are the most appropriate to ensure community engagement in such efforts. As professionals, social workers engage in direct roles, intermediary roles and macro-level roles to deliver the best health outcomes (Ruth & Marshall, 2017). In the case of NTDs, since the role of social determinants is evident and since NTD programmes require community engagement, social workers can play a pivotal role. By advocating for health equity, engaging communities, addressing social determinants and collaborating with healthcare professionals, social workers can contribute significantly to the broader efforts in mitigating the impact of NTDs on vulnerable populations. Social work's historical commitment to public health underscores the potential for positive change in the fight against these diseases. The following chapters in this book discuss the need to establish NTD social work in effective and sustainable interventions for elimination and control.

1.7 Conclusion

This chapter sheds light on the intricate interplay between NTD burden and social factors. NTDs are a prime example of global health disparities, reflecting systemic issues in resource allocation and attention. These diseases inflict individual suffering and perpetuate adverse outcomes for entire communities, necessitating a holistic approach beyond traditional disease-specific frameworks. Addressing NTDs requires multifaceted strategies that consider environmental, social and economic factors, with socio-economic factors emerging as a critical determinant, intertwining with NTD infection in a cyclical manner. Moreover, cultural and behavioural factors influence NTD transmission, highlighting the importance of promoting healthy practices such as water, sanitation and hygiene (WASH). Despite progress in understanding and addressing NTDs, challenges persist. Social workers, with their expertise in health equity and community mobilisation, can contribute to sustainable interventions for NTD control and elimination, and the following chapters build upon the social nature of NTDs to argue for the case of NTD social work.

References

Ackley, C., Elsheikh, M., & Zaman, S. (2021). Scoping review of neglected tropical disease interventions and health promotion: A framework for successful NTD interventions as evidenced by the literature. *PLoS Neglected Tropical Diseases, 15*(7), e0009278. https://doi.org/10.1371/journal.pntd.0009278

Arcaya, M. C., Arcaya, A. L., & Subramanian, S. V. (2015). Inequalities in health: Definitions, concepts, and theories. *Global Health Action, 8*, 27106. https://doi.org/10.3402/gha.v8.27106

Bishwajit, G., Ide, S., & Ghosh, S. (2014). Social determinants of infectious diseases in South Asia. *International Scholarly Research Notices, 2014*, 135243. https://doi.org/10.1155/2014/135243

Booth, M. (2018). Climate change and the neglected tropical diseases. *Advances in Parasitology, 100*, 39–126. https://doi.org/10.1016/bs.apar.2018.02.001

Chris, B., Singh, S., & Sudarshi, D. (2011). Neglected tropical diseases, conflict, and the right to health. In E. R. Choffness & D. A. Relman (Eds.), *The causes and impacts of neglected tropical and zoonotic diseases: Opportunities for integrated intervention strategies*. National Academies Press. Available from: https://www.ncbi.nlm.nih.gov/books/NBK62508/

De Rycker, M., Baragaña, B., Duce, S. L., & Gilbert, I. H. (2018). Challenges and recent progress in drug discovery for tropical diseases. *Nature, 559*(7715), 498–506.

Degarege, A., Erko, B., Negash, Y., & Animut, A. (2022). Intestinal helminth infection, anemia, undernutrition and academic performance among school children in northwestern Ethiopia. *Microorganisms, 10*(7), 1353. https://doi.org/10.3390/microorganisms10071353

Deribe, K. (2015). Neglected tropical disease targets must include morbidity. *The Lancet. Global Health, 3*(10), e596. https://doi.org/10.1016/S2214-109X(15)00185-0

Fee, E., & Gonzalez, A. R. (2017). The history of health equity: Concept and vision. *Diversity and Equality in Health and Care, 14*(3), 148–152.

Garchitorena, A., Sokolow, S. H., Roche, B., Ngonghala, C. N., Jocque, M., Lund, A., Barry, M., Mordecai, E. A., Daily, G. C., Jones, J. H., Andrews, J. R., Bendavid, E., Luby, S. P., LaBeaud, A. D., Seetah, K., Guegan, J. F., Bonds, M. H., & De Leo, G. A. (2017). Disease ecology, health and the environment: A framework to account for ecological and socio-economic drivers in the control of neglected tropical diseases. *Philosophical Transactions of the Royal Society B: Biological Sciences, 372*(1722), 20160128.

George, N. S., David, S. C., Nabiryo, M., Sunday, B. A., Olanrewaju, O. F., Yangaza, Y., & Shomuyiwa, D. O. (2023). Addressing neglected tropical diseases in Africa: A health equity perspective. *Global Health Research and Policy, 8*(1), 30.

Halim, A. F. N. A., Ahmad, D., Miaw Yn, J. L., Masdor, N. A., Ramly, N., Othman, R., Kandayah, T., Hassan, M. R., & Dapari, R. (2022). Factors associated with the acceptability of mass drug Administration for Filariasis: A systematic review. *International Journal of Environmental Research and Public Health, 19*(19), 12971. https://doi.org/10.3390/ijerph191912971

Herricks, J. R., Hotez, P. J., Wanga, V., Coffeng, L. E., Haagsma, J. A., Basáñez, M. G., et al. (2017). The global burden of disease study 2013: What does it mean for the NTDs? *PLoS Neglected Tropical Diseases, 11*(8), e0005424.

Hill, S. (2016). Axes of health inequalities and intersectionality. In K. E. Smith, C. Bambra, & S. E. Hill (Eds.), *Health inequalities: Critical perspectives* (pp. 209–213). Oxford University Press.

Hotez, P. (2009). Mass drug administration and integrated control for the world's high-prevalence neglected tropical diseases. *Clinical Pharmacology & Therapeutics, 85*(6), 659–664.

Hotez, P. J. (2014). Ten global "hotspots" for the neglected tropical diseases. *PLoS Neglected Tropical Diseases, 8*(5), e2496.

Hotez, P. J. (2021). *Forgotten people, forgotten diseases: The neglected tropical diseases and their impact on global health and development*. Wiley.

Hotez, P. J., & Lo, N. C. (2020). Neglected tropical diseases: Public health control programs and mass drug administration. In E. T. Ryan, D. R. Hill, T. Solomon, N. Aronson, & T. P. Endy (Eds.), *Hunter's tropical medicine and emerging infectious diseases* (pp. 209–213). Elsevier.

Hotez, P. J., Bottazzi, M. E., Franco-Paredes, C., Ault, S. K., & Periago, M. R. (2008). The neglected tropical diseases of Latin America and the Caribbean: A review of disease burden and distribution and a roadmap for control and elimination. *PLoS Neglected Tropical Diseases, 2*(9), e300. https://doi.org/10.1371/journal.pntd.0000300

Hotez, P. J., Savioli, L., & Fenwick, A. (2012). Neglected tropical diseases of the Middle East and North Africa: Review of their prevalence, distribution, and opportunities for control. *PLoS Neglected Tropical Diseases, 6*(2), e1475. https://doi.org/10.1371/journal.pntd.0001475

Hotez, P. J., Aksoy, S., Brindley, P. J., & Kamhawi, S. (2020). What constitutes a neglected tropical disease? *PLoS Neglected Tropical Diseases, 14*(1), e0008001. https://doi.org/10.1371/journal.pntd.0008001

Houweling, T. A., Karim-Kos, H. E., Kulik, M. C., Stolk, W. A., Haagsma, J. A., Lenk, E. J., Richardus, J. H., & de Vlas, S. J. (2016). Socioeconomic inequalities in neglected tropical diseases: A systematic review. *PLoS Neglected Tropical Diseases, 10*(5), e0004546. https://doi.org/10.1371/journal.pntd.0004546

Jung, Y. L., Hwang, J., & Yoo, H. S. (2020). Disease burden metrics and the innovations of leading pharmaceutical companies: A global and regional comparative study. *Globalization and Health, 16*(1), 1–11.

Kemmerling, U., Osuna, A., Schijman, A. G., & Truyens, C. (2019). Congenital transmission of Trypanosoma cruzi: A review about the interactions between the parasite, the placenta, the maternal and the fetal/neonatal immune responses. *Frontiers in Microbiology, 10*, 1854.

Kuper, H. (2019). Neglected tropical diseases and disability-what is the link? *Transactions of the Royal Society of Tropical Medicine and Hygiene, 113*(12), 839–844. https://doi.org/10.1093/trstmh/trz001

Lobo, D. A., Velayudhan, R., Chatterjee, P., Kohli, H., & Hotez, P. J. (2011). The neglected tropical diseases of India and South Asia: Review of their prevalence, distribution, and control or elimination. *PLoS Neglected Tropical Diseases, 5*(10), e1222. https://doi.org/10.1371/journal.pntd.0001222

Madon, S., Malecela, M. N., Mashoto, K., Donohue, R., Mubyazi, G., & Michael, E. (2018). The role of community participation for sustainable integrated neglected tropical diseases and water, sanitation and hygiene intervention programs: A pilot project in Tanzania. *Social Science & Medicine (1982), 202*, 28–37. https://doi.org/10.1016/j.socscimed.2018.02.016

Manyeh, A. K., Ibisomi, L., Ramaswamy, R., Baiden, F., & Chirwa, T. (2020). Exploring factors affecting quality implementation of lymphatic filariasis mass drug administration in bole and central Gonja districts in northern Ghana. *PLoS Neglected Tropical Diseases, 14*(8), e0007009. https://doi.org/10.1371/journal.pntd.0007009

Marchal, B., Van Dormael, M., Pirard, M., Cavalli, A., Kegels, G., & Polman, K. (2011). Neglected tropical disease (NTD) control in health systems: The interface between programmes and general health services. *Acta Tropica, 120*, S177–S185.

Meltsner, M. (1966). Equality and health. *University of Pennsylvania Law Review, 115*(1), 22–38.

Mitra, A. K., & Mawson, A. R. (2017). Neglected tropical diseases: Epidemiology and global burden. *Tropical Medicine and Infectious Disease, 2*(3), 36.

Molyneux, D. H., Hotez, P. J., & Fenwick, A. (2005). "Rapid-impact interventions": How a policy of integrated control for Africa's neglected tropical diseases could benefit the poor. *PLoS Medicine, 2*(11), e336.

Ness, T. E., Agrawal, V., Bedard, K., Ouellette, L., Erickson, T. A., Hotez, P., & Weatherhead, J. E. (2020). Maternal hookworm infection and its effects on maternal health: A systematic review and meta-analysis. *The American Journal of Tropical Medicine and Hygiene, 103*(5), 1958–1968. https://doi.org/10.4269/ajtmh.20-0503

Ochola, E. A., Karanja, D. M. S., & Elliott, S. J. (2021). The impact of neglected tropical diseases (NTDs) on health and wellbeing in sub-Saharan Africa (SSA): A case study of Kenya. *PLoS Neglected Tropical Diseases, 15*(2), e0009131. https://doi.org/10.1371/journal.pntd.0009131

Ochola, E. A., Karanja, D. M., & Elliott, S. J. (2022). Local tips, global impact: Community-driven measures as avenues of promoting inclusion in the control of neglected tropical diseases: A case study in Kenya. *Infectious Diseases of Poverty, 11*(04), 81–90.

Parke, S., Dauda, N., & Ayarza, R. (2022). Behaviour insight shadowing: Examining daily life settings for the prevention of neglected tropical disease. *International Health, 14*(Supplement_2), ii25–ii32. https://doi.org/10.1093/inthealth/ihac042

Pastrana, N. A., Beran, D., Somerville, C., Heller, O., Correia, J. C., & Suggs, L. S. (2020). The process of building the priority of neglected tropical diseases: A global policy analysis. *PLoS Neglected Tropical Diseases, 14*(8), e0008498. https://doi.org/10.1371/journal.pntd.0008498

Peterson, J. K., Bakuza, J., & Standley, C. J. (2020). One health and neglected tropical diseases-multisectoral solutions to endemic challenges. *Tropical Medicine and Infectious Disease, 6*(1), 4. https://doi.org/10.3390/tropicalmed6010004

Raheel, U., Faheem, M., Riaz, M. N., Kanwal, N., Javed, F., & Qadri, I. (2011). Dengue fever in the Indian subcontinent: An overview. *The Journal of Infection in Developing Countries, 5*(04), 239–247.

Ruth, B. J., & Marshall, J. W. (2017). A history of social work in public health. *American Journal of Public Health, 107*(S3), S236–S242. https://doi.org/10.2105/AJPH.2017.304005

Singh, S. K. (Ed.). (2017). *Neglected tropical diseases-South Asia*. Springer International Publishing.

Wagstaff, A. (2002). Poverty and health sector inequalities. *Bulletin of the World Health Organization, 80*(2), 97–105.
Warusavithana, S., Atta, H., Osman, M., & Hutin, Y. (2022). Review of the neglected tropical diseases programme implementation during 2012–2019 in the WHO-Eastern Mediterranean region. *PLoS Neglected Tropical Diseases, 16*(9), e0010665. https://doi.org/10.1371/journal.pntd.0010665
WHO. (1946). *Constitution of the World Health Organization*. Retrieved from https://treaties.un.org/doc/Treaties/1948/04/19480407%2010-51%20PM/Ch_IX_01p.pdf
WHO. (2020). *Regional action framework for control and elimination of neglected tropical diseases in the Western Pacific*. Retrieved from https://www.eliminateschisto.org/sites/gsa/files/content/attachments/2020-05-28/WHOWPR_Regiona_Action_Framework_NTDs.pdf
WHO. (2023, June 1). *Lymphatic filariasis*. Retrieved from https://www.who.int/news-room/fact-sheets/detail/lymphatic-filariasis#:~:text=When%20lymphatic%20filariasis%20develops%20into,and%20hydrocele%20(scrotal%20swelling)
WHO. (n.d.). *Neglected tropical diseases*. Retrieved from https://www.who.int/health-topics/neglected-tropical-diseases#tab=tab_1
World Health Organization. (2012). *Accelerating work to overcome the global impact of neglected tropical diseases: A roadmap for implementation* (No. WHO/HTM/NTD/2012.5). World Health Organization.
World Health Organization. (2015). *Water sanitation & hygiene for accelerating and sustaining progress on neglected tropical diseases: A global strategy 2015–2020* (No. WHO/FWC/WSH/15.12). World Health Organization.
World Health Organization. (2020). *Ending the neglect to attain the sustainable development goals: A road map for neglected tropical diseases 2021–2030*. Retrieved from https://iris.who.int/handle/10665/332094
Yajima, A., Lin, Z., Mohamed, A. J., Dash, A. P., & Rijal, S. (2023). Finishing the task of eliminating neglected tropical diseases (NTDs) in WHO South-East Asia region: Promises kept, challenges, and the way forward. *The Lancet Regional Health-Southeast Asia, 18*, 1–11. https://doi.org/10.1016/j.lansea.2023.100302
Yao, Q., Li, X., Luo, F., Yang, L., Liu, C., & Sun, J. (2019). The historical roots and seminal research on health equity: A referenced publication year spectroscopy (RPYS) analysis. *International Journal for Equity in Health, 18*, 1–15.

Chapter 2
Neglected Tropical Diseases and the Social Dimension of Illness in India

2.1 Introduction

This chapter unearths the social dimension of neglected tropical diseases (NTDs) and discusses how marginalised communities are disproportionately vulnerable to NTDs due to their socioeconomic position, making the subject matter a question of health inequity. The intersectional disadvantages experienced by specific communities in India that make them vulnerable to NTDs are discussed in this chapter. The overall aim is to establish the reciprocal relationship between poverty and NTDs, disproportionately affecting certain groups in an endless cycle, leading to endemic areas. In addition, the chapter examines the long-term consequences of NTDs on the affected communities, shedding light on the potential for prolonged marginalisation and its impact on their socio-economic well-being.

2.2 Towards Understanding NTDs and Social Dimension of Illness: A Conceptual Map

In India, the prevailing approaches for understanding neglected tropical diseases (NTDs) primarily consider environmental variables (Faust et al., 2018), neglecting the significant impact of socio-economic and behavioural dimensions of affected communities. While NTDs indeed show a robust association with environmental parameters like temperature, land cover and usage pattern and topographic conditions, it is crucial to acknowledge the substantial impact of social dimensions on the spread of this group of diseases, especially in the unique context of India. Previous research has documented a strong association between people's lifestyle, quality of life and their interaction with the environment with major NTDs like dengue,

© The Author(s), under exclusive license to Springer Nature Switzerland AG 2024

M. Jabir, A. C. Choolayil, *Social Work with Populations Vulnerable to Neglected Tropical Diseases*, SpringerBriefs in Social Work,
https://doi.org/10.1007/978-3-031-68997-0_2

filariasis and leishmaniasis (Aagaard-Hansen & Chaignat, 2010; Bhutta et al., 2014). In light of this, the section explores the social dimensions of NTDs in India by addressing prevalent social conditions such as poverty, social inequality, housing and sanitation conditions, work environments, cultural aspects and healthcare accessibility. To elucidate this, we have developed a framework utilising key variables identified in the literature and presented in Fig. 2.1.

The social dimension of NTDs is structured around two primary influencing factors: poverty and social identity. Poverty contributes to NTD prevalence in various ways, including financial problems in accessing healthcare, engagement in disease-vulnerable occupations, unsafe housing and sanitation, urbanisation-related challenges, limited educational opportunities and malnutrition. Social identity and cultural factors further shape the NTD landscape, with considerations such as ethnicity, caste dynamics, social stigma attached to NTDs, adherence to social norms and customs, and reliance on traditional healing practices impacting disease transmission and management. Furthermore, some intermediary factors play a significant role in mediating the relationship between influencing factors and NTD outcomes. These factors are categorised into three groups: environmental and vector-pathogen-related factors, behavioural factors, and health system-related factors. Environmental factors such as geography, temperature and vector density influence disease transmission, while behavioural factors like individual lifestyle choices, usage of preventive measures, water storage practices, treatment-seeking behaviours and population movements between disease endemic and non-endemic regions affect NTD spread. Additionally, health system-related factors encompass the status of healthcare accessibility, health financing by the government, disease surveillance capabilities, supply chain management, policy frameworks and leadership effectiveness, all of which influence NTD control efforts. Ultimately, the

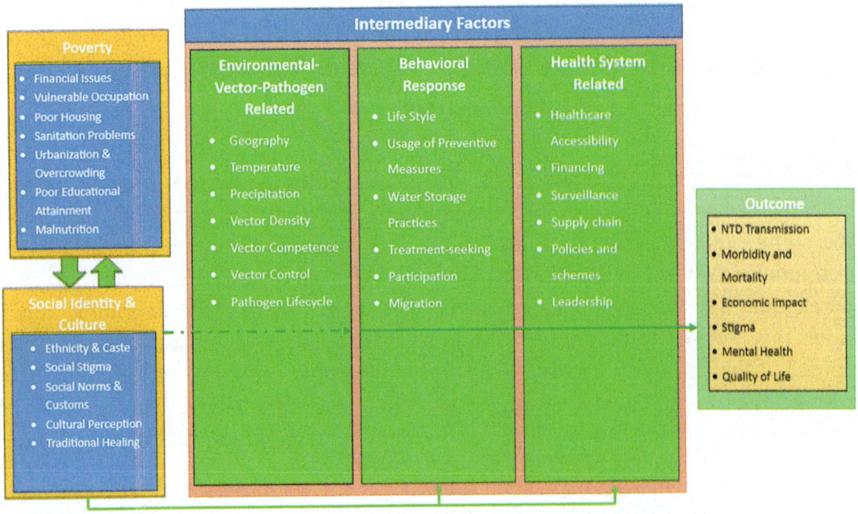

Fig. 2.1 Conceptual map

outcomes of these complex interactions manifest in various forms, including NTD transmission rates, related morbidity and mortality, economic repercussions in communities, social stigma, mental health implications and overall quality of life of affected communities.

2.3 NTDs and Vicious Cycle of Poverty

Poverty, often defined as a deficiency in financial resources with negative societal repercussions (Sen, 1983), is closely intertwined with social inequality, characterised by persistent disparities in the distributions of goods, wealth, opportunities, rewards and punishments within a group or society. The economic hardships stemming from poverty and prejudices linked to social inequality significantly impact a person's lifestyle choices, consumption habits, social interactions, and, most importantly, their health outcomes and well-being.

It has been widely reported that poverty is a significant factor contributing to the prevalence of NTDs across various countries (Aagaard-Hansen & Chaignat, 2010). NTDs are prevalent in regions characterised by low human development index (HDI), socio-economic disparities, discrimination and poverty (Hotez et al., 2014). Evidently, NTDs disproportionately affect poor and vulnerable populations, primarily in Africa, Asia, Latin America and the Caribbean regions (WHO, 2017). The regions with the largest NTD burden are Sub-Saharan Africa and South Asia, where poverty and inequalities prevail. Studies conducted across various countries indicated that NTDs are particularly prevalent among underprivileged people living in resource-constrained settings, where disease-transmitting vectors are abundant (Williams et al., 2023).

NTDs often perpetuate a vicious cycle of poverty, exacerbating the socio-economic disparities (Magalhães et al., 2023). Figure 2.2 depicts a multifaceted cycle wherein poverty serves as the initial catalyst, leading to a cascade of interconnected consequences. Poor housing and sanitation conditions in impoverished areas arising from poverty elevate the risk of exposure to neglected tropical diseases (NTDs), which are further exacerbated by malnutrition due to inadequate access to healthcare and nutritious food. For instance, a family living in a slum with limited access to safe housing and clean water may be at higher risk of contracting vector-borne diseases due to stagnant water in the surrounding areas and a greater number of breeding sources in and around the houses. This heightened susceptibility to NTDs results in increased morbidity, impairing cognitive development and physical health, consequently hindering educational attainment and reducing productivity. As a result, family members fall ill frequently, leading to increased medical expenses and decreased productivity. Previous studies found that NTDs affect lower-income households, resulting in low productivity, disability and social stigma (Bhutta et al., 2014). Additionally, the lack of proper nutrition due to financial constraints further weakens their immune systems, making them more susceptible to infections. The resultant low income due to productivity issues perpetuates the cycle of poverty,

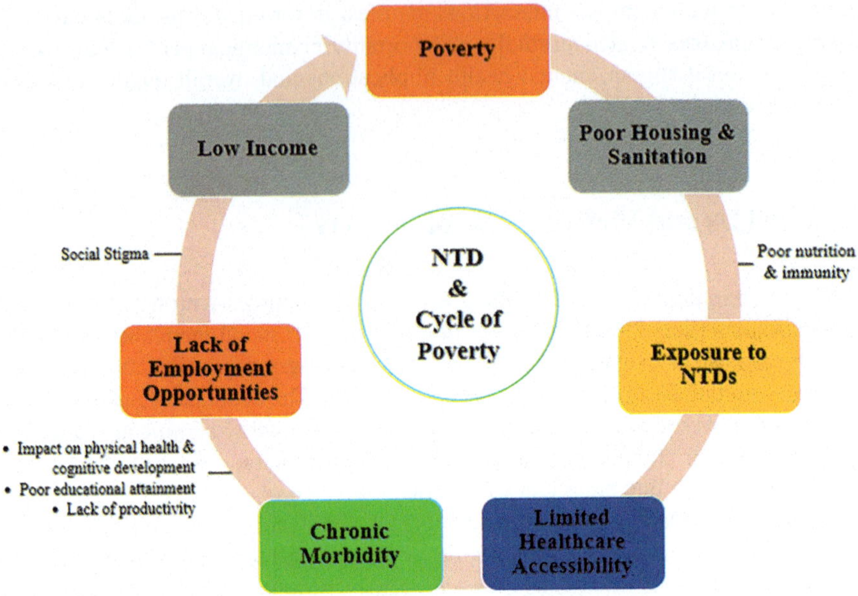

Fig. 2.2 NTD and cycle of poverty

while social stigma further marginalises affected individuals, ultimately leading back to poverty. This cyclical relationship underscores the intricate web of factors entwining poverty and NTDs.

2.4 Poverty as a Pervasive Catalyst for NTDs in India

Like many other countries, poverty plays a significant role in the prevalence of neglected tropical diseases in India. Communities with poor living standards residing in impoverished regions bear a disproportionately higher burden of illness (Hotez et al., 2014). A notable example is lymphatic filariasis (LF), which stands as one of the most debilitating NTDs in India, constituting 40% of global cases and affecting around 670 million people across 256 districts (Tripathi et al., 2022). The disease has historically been associated with poverty, underdevelopment and inadequate sanitation in various regions of the country. Most evidently, the LF "transmission hotspots" are located in small rural settlements with poor access to economic resources and substandard sanitary conditions (Swaminathan et al., 2012). The common mosquito vector for LF is *Cx. quinquefasciatus*, which prevails in overcrowded areas inhabited by disadvantaged communities facing poor housing and drainage conditions (Modi et al., 2021).

Research examining factors related to LF in India consistently found higher infection risks among individuals residing in economically deprived areas compared to their wealthier counterparts. For instance, a study conducted in Andhra Pradesh reported nearly twice the prevalence of *Wuchereria bancrofti* microfilaria among residents in poor villages (4.9%) and impoverished urban neighbourhoods (1.3%) compared to wealthier ones. It has been reported that the substandard housing and inadequate sanitation facilities stemming from poverty created a condition that is conducive to the proliferation of disease-causing mosquito vectors in the region (Mutheneni et al., 2016; Upadhyayula et al., 2012). In contrast, the higher and middle-income groups of people generally benefit from cleaner homes and facilities, enabling them to maintain a safer environment from these diseases.

This trend extends to other NTDs such as dengue, visceral leishmaniasis (VL), chikungunya, leprosy and soil-transmitted helminths (STH) as well. Dengue research in India often highlighted that the disease is linked to poor environmental hygiene due to resource constraints, facilitating the rapid spread of the disease in various urban and rural settings in the country (Telle et al., 2016). Supporting this argument, a large-scale dengue burden study among 17930 individuals in India found that 43.6% of the infected belong to the poverty line (BPL) category (Murhekar et al., 2019). In addition, a hospital-based study by Nayak et al. (2021), carried out between 2017 and 2018 in Odisha, found a significant disease burden among patients from poor economic backgrounds, reflecting that 54% of patients were from lower socio-economic strata. Regarding the urban cases of dengue, the absence or irregular supply of water and the subsequent need for water storage among disadvantaged communities, especially those living in slums and underdeveloped areas, create ideal breeding sites for dengue-causing *Aedes* mosquitoes. The regions with the poorest water access and poverty have been found to have the highest proportion of containers positive for mosquitoes (Telle et al., 2016). Similarly, in the case of Chikungunya, another NTD caused by the same *Aedes* mosquito, poverty was found to be an important determinant for the spread of the disease (Kumar et al., 2007). Research has demonstrated that individuals with improper toilet facilities and engaged open defecation have a higher likelihood of CHIKV in the country (Paulson et al., 2022).

Visceral leishmaniasis (VL), or Kala Azar, is one of the major NTDs in India caused by a parasite belonging to *Leishmania donovani*. The disease is mostly found among poor rural communities in the northern region of the country (Sundar et al., 2018). The individual-level studies carried out in Bihar and West Bengal have consistently reported a strong association between poverty and the incidence of VL, as the majority of the affected households belong to the below poverty line (BPL) (Guha et al., 2020). Moreover, the odds of VL infection have been reported to be 1.6–3.4 times higher compared to the middle and higher socio-economic classes (Bhunia et al., 2012). Similarly, a high prevalence of STH is reported among children from socio-economically deprived and poorer households in the country, indicating a broader impact of poverty on these diseases (Houweling et al., 2016). In addition, systematic reviews on leprosy highlighted the disease's association with the social dimension of individuals, such as those living in overcrowded households and engaged in manual labour (Pescarini et al., 2018). The majority of the leprosy cases in the country are reported to people from poor socio-economic status (Alam et al., 1998). Overall, these findings underscore the complex interplay between poverty and neglected tropical diseases in India.

2.4.1 *Poor Sanitation and Substandard Housing: A Nexus to NTDs*

Housing and sanitation facilities are often considered outcomes of better economic positions and opportunities within a community. Poverty serves as a fundamental driver of substandard housing and poorer sanitation facilities in India, exposing millions of individuals to the risk of NTDs in the country. According to the 76th round of the National Sample Survey (NSS) in 2019, approximately 25% of the households in rural India reside in kutcha houses, while 30% lack access to latrine facilities, 39% lack a drainage system and 48.1% dispose of household wastewater untreated in open and low-lying areas or streets (Government of India, 2019). Additionally, around 6.5 crore people live in slum areas without adequate sanitation facilities. Inadequate waste management and open defecation are prevalent in many parts of the country (Saleem et al., 2019). These circumstances act as major push factors, creating an environment conducive to the proliferation of disease vectors and the transmission of NTDs. For instance, the bancroftian filariasis is widespread in the country, with the primary vector, *Cx. Quinquefasciatus* breeds in locations lacking basic sanitary conditions. In the case of STH, poor sanitation, coupled with the absence of footwear-wearing habits, significantly impacts the disease prevalence (Salam & Azam, 2017). Similarly, VL is primarily found in poor settlements in the states of Bihar, West Bengal and Uttar Pradesh, where housing and sanitation facilities are lacking (WHO, 2024).

Furthermore, large-scale entomological surveys conducted in India have revealed that poorly constructed houses exhibit higher vector densities than well-constructed houses (Nguela et al., 2020; Perry et al., 2013a, b). Individuals residing in huts, thatched and tiled houses are at a significantly higher risk of contracting dengue and chikungunya in comparison to those residing in concrete-constructed structures (Swain et al., 2020). This underscores the critical role of housing conditions in the transmission dynamics of NTDs within the country. The risk is further amplified due to factors like poor ventilation due to substandard construction and increased carbon dioxide levels resulting from overcrowding, thereby exacerbating the susceptibility of residents in impoverished settlements to NTD infections (Upadhyayula et al., 2012). Further, specific risk factors associated with VL include the presence of houses with mud walls, dampness in houses and the proximity of peri-domestic vegetation, which serve as conducive environments for the survival and proliferation of insect vectors (Bern et al., 2010). These findings indicate the complex dynamics of poverty, housing and sanitation in the spread of NTDs in India. Therefore, controlling these diseases underlining requires targeted interventions addressing housing conditions and sanitation to mitigate disease transmission effectively.

2.4.2 *Urbanisation and the Spread of NTDs in India*

Rapid urbanisation has significant implications for the rise of NTDs (Hotez, 2017). India has been witnessing substantial urban growth in recent years, with the urban population increasing from 286 million in 2001 to 377 million in 2011 (Bhagat, 2018). The World Urbanization Prospects report by the UN Department of Economic and Social Affairs (UN DESA) in 2018 indicated that future increases in the world's urban population are expected to be highly concentrated in just a few countries, including India, China and Nigeria. By 2050, India is projected to have added 416 million urban dwellers.

The expansion of urbanisation is often associated with the emergence and spread of NTDs, as favourable conditions for the vectors are created (Kolimenakis et al., 2021). It becomes evident that a growing number of areas around the globe are becoming increasingly vulnerable to the spread of vectors and diseases due to rapid and unplanned urbanisation, compounded by other socio-ecological challenges, including climate and environmental change (Campbell-Lendrum et al., 2015).

NTDs, indeed in India, have been significantly influenced by the rapid urbanisation occurring in the country in the last few years. For instance, rapid urbanisation has led to a higher prevalence of dengue and rabies. In India, the incidence of rabies is 59% in urban areas, mostly due to overcrowding (Nair et al., 2016). Urban areas with high population density provide a larger pool of hosts for vector mosquitoes to feed on, facilitating the rapid spread of NTDs. This is particularly problematic in informal settlements or slums where overcrowding is common. Reports shows that approximately 18% of urban households in the country lived in slums in 2011 (Chandramouli, 2011). The living conditions of the urban poor are characterised by a high-density of population, unhygienic shelter, substandard sanitation facilities, and poor drainage and solid waste disposal. Residents of slums typically have limited access to healthcare services also, which hinders timely diagnosis and treatment of diseases. This delay can lead to more severe health outcomes and higher transmission rates. Addressing these challenges requires improving urban planning, enhancing public health infrastructure and implementing effective disease prevention programs.

2.4.3 *Poverty, Vulnerable Occupations and NTD Risk*

Occupation, a vital element of the social dimension, goes beyond mere economic sustenance. For many, occupation is not just a means of earning but also an integral part of their culture, social identity and social structure. The occupational choices of individuals are closely linked to their socioeconomic status in society. For instance, engaging in occupations such as agriculture, manual labour, street vending, sewage work, fishing, etc., often characterises the livelihoods of economically disadvantaged individuals. The caste system, particularly in rural India, is closely intertwined with occupational status, with Dalits predominantly found in less-paid occupations and manual labour works (Gang et al., 2017).

The linkage between poverty and occupational status has been extensively explored in the literature and revolves around the degree to which the income earned enables one to access essential goods and services. There is a strong association between social inequality and occupation as unequal access to employment opportunities in the labour market (ILO, 2008).

Occupation is closely connected to individual health outcomes, particularly regarding NTDs in India. Evidence suggests the undeniable influence of occupation on shaping the prevalence and distribution of NTDs among diverse communities in the country. For instance, individuals employed in agriculture and allied fields exhibit a significant correlation with the prevalence of certain NTDs, such as leptospirosis, Japanese encephalitis and scrub typhus, due to the proliferation of vectors and proximity (Erlanger et al., 2005). Leptospirosis is considered a significant NTD in India, contributing to acute febrile illness. The bacteria responsible for the disease *Leptospira* genus follow a transmission cycle facilitated by the presence of urine from infected domestic rodents. Typically, people working in rural settings and involved in agriculture bear a disproportionate burden of this disease (Prist et al., 2016). The seroprevalence of leptospirosis is high among specific groups such as sewage workers, hospital sanitary workers and fishermen (Tullu & Karande, 2009). Similarly, the prevalence of ascariasis and hookworm infections has been found to be significantly high among tea-picking communities (Traub et al., 2004; Galgamuwa et al., 2018). Furthermore, agricultural laborers and cattle owners face an increased risk of visceral leishmaniasis (VL) (Bern et al., 2010). As mentioned earlier, individuals from disadvantaged communities and economically poor backgrounds are often engaged in such occupations, making them more susceptible to these diseases.

2.4.4 *Educational Attainment: A Key Determinant in NTD Prevalence*

Education holds a pivotal place in the social dimensions of India, given the significant correlation between an individual's educational attainment and their social status. Additionally, there exists a distinct relationship between education and poverty, with nations having inadequate educational systems tending to experience a higher prevalence of poverty. UNESCO global education monitoring report, 2019, indicated that offering two or more years of education to every adult or ensuring the completion of secondary schooling could potentially lift 420 million people out of poverty. In India, previous research has consistently established a close association between the educational status of individuals and the prevalence of NTDs. For instance, a country-wide dengue burden study conducted by Murhekar et al. (2019) revealed that nearly 44% of individuals testing positive for IgG antibodies against dengue had completed only primary school education, and 8.2% had received no formal education. Similarly, Paulson et al. (2022) found that dengue and chikungunya infection risk is lower among those with high school education and above. It implies that individuals with less education may be more susceptible to contracting dengue and chikungunya, possibly due to factors such as limited knowledge of the disease, including symptoms and preventive measures.

Furthermore, research on other NTDs, such as VL and STH, also found that the level of education attained by individuals plays a significant role in their susceptibility to the disease in India. For instance, a study conducted by Perry et al. in 2013a, b identified that individuals with lower levels of education were at higher risk of contracting VL. Additionally, a study examining intestinal helminthiasis among schoolchildren by Wani and Ahmad (2009) further illustrates these dynamics. They found a notably high prevalence of intestinal helminthiasis among children whose mothers were illiterate. This finding suggests that the educational status of parents may influence hygiene practices, access to healthcare and overall health literacy within households, thereby impacting the risk of parasitic infections among children. These studies highlight the complex interplay between education and NTD prevalence in the country. They underscore the importance of addressing educational disparities and promoting health education initiatives to reduce the burden of NTDs and improve overall public health outcomes.

2.5 Social Identity in NTD Landscape in India

An individual's social identity includes many components, such as gender, race, ethnicity and sexual orientation, which often intersect with health outcomes. In India, caste, religion, gender and ethnicity are significant social identities (Dasgupta et al., 2023), profoundly influencing various aspects of individuals' lives, including their access to resources, opportunities and health outcomes. Social identity, especially caste, has been found to be one of the relevant indicators for the health and well-being of individuals in the country (Baru et al., 2010).

In India, the significance of caste and community identities continues to play a significant role in shaping NTD outcomes. It becomes evident in the clustering of certain NTDs within specific hamlets or areas predominantly inhabited by particular castes or social groups. A significant proportion of VL cases are concentrated in hamlets primarily occupied by Scheduled Castes or Scheduled Tribes. Approximately 80% of documented VL cases were reported from these marginalised communities (Priyamvada et al., 2021). Similarly, scabies is a major global public health problem and affect close to 130 million people worldwide. In India, the burden of scabies is particularly high in various tribal communities, ranging from 8.4% to 20.6% (Behera et al., 2021).

Marginalised communities such as SCs and STs have been historically subjected to social and economic marginalisation (Raghavendra, 2020). These communities often face challenges such as poverty, limited access to education and healthcare, and discrimination, all of which contribute to their vulnerability to NTDs. These communities often reside in areas with poor infrastructure, inadequate housing and limited access to clean water and sanitation facilities, which are conducive to the breeding of disease vectors such as sandflies, the carriers of the VL parasite. Additionally, socioeconomic factors such as poverty and malnutrition prevalent in these communities can weaken immune systems, making individuals more susceptible to infections like VL. Furthermore, historical and social inequalities, including caste-based discrimination and stigmatisation, may also contribute to the higher vulnerability of these groups to NTDs.

2.6 Culture: Shaping Health Belief and Treatment Decisions for NTDs

Cultural beliefs and practices play a significant role in shaping how individuals perceive and interpret illness, influencing their approaches to healthcare. Different cultures may have distinct views on health, the causes of diseases and appropriate treatments. NTDs such as lymphatic filariasis and leprosy have been endemic in several Indian villages for decades, and the local perception of these diseases, including their names and causes, varies widely across regions in the country. Cultural interpretation often views these diseases with a supernatural lens, with some attributing them to impure blood, past sin, hereditary problems or divine curses (Datta et al., 2022).

Moreover, social and cultural factors significantly influence the decision of patients and their families regarding treatment-seeking behaviours and acceptance of medical interventions (Mandal & Saha, 2015). For instance, Stephen et al. (2014) highlighted how societal norms and social stigma surrounding NTDs create barriers to accessing healthcare services, leading to delayed diagnosis and treatment initiation. In addition, traditional healing practices, folk medicine and magico-religious practices remain prevalent in many Indian communities, especially in NTD endemic settings, as alternative approaches to manage diseases (Jacob & Franco-Paredes, 2008), which have been found as one of the major risk factors for delay in seeking appropriate diagnosis and treatment.

The nexus of cultural beliefs, social norms and healthcare practices profoundly influences the management of NTDs in India. Recognising the diversity of cultural perspectives and addressing societal stigma and misconceptions are pivotal in ensuring effective prevention, diagnosis and treatment of NTDs. Efforts to combat NTDs in India must acknowledge and engage with local belief systems, fostering partnerships between traditional healers, community leaders and modern healthcare providers.

2.7 Behavioural Determinants in NTD Transmission

Individual behaviour is intricately intertwined with the social structure, norms and socialisation processes within a society. The social structure of a society provides the foundation upon which behavioural patterns are established. Behavioural factors significantly influence the transmission and control of NTDs in India. A wide range of practices and actions that individuals undertake in their daily lives, including hygiene practices, usage of preventive measures, treatment-seeking behaviour, knowledge and attitude, play a pivotal role.

Personal hygiene behaviours, such as handwashing, sanitation practices and waste disposal, are fundamental in preventing the transmission of NTDs. For instance, inadequate sanitation and contaminated water sources contribute to diseases like STH, filariasis and dengue. For NTDs such as LF and leprosy, having a hygienic environment lowers the chances of opportunistic infections by reducing exposure to pathogens (Garsed & Waite, 2015). To improve hygiene, steps like ending open defecation and preventing human waste from entering surroundings, as well as regular cleaning and disinfection of surfaces, can be taken.

Most of the NTDs can be prevented through the consistent use of suggested precautionary measures against the vectors and pathogens. For instance, taking drugs during MDA campaigns, usage of insecticide-treated bed nets and environmental cleanliness can reduce the risk of LF. Similarly, VL can be prevented using LLINs, insecticides, destruction of sandfly breeding grounds and insecticidal dog collars. For STH infections, prevention is possible through the reduction of faecal contamination of soil by avoiding open defecation and hygiene measures through washing hands and proper food preparation.

Prompt recognition of symptoms and seeking timely medical care are some of the important proactive behaviours against NTDs. Delayed treatment-seeking behaviour may exacerbate the progression of NTDs, leading to increased morbidity and mortality rates. For instance, delays in diagnosis and treatment of dengue lead to an expanded dengue syndrome (EDS), among some high-risk groups such as pregnant women, infants, the elderly and patients with coronary artery disease (Trivedi & Chakravarty, 2022). The behavioural outcomes are often influenced by the education and awareness of the disease and preventive measures. So, increasing knowledge about disease transmission, symptoms and preventive measures empowers individuals to make informed decisions regarding their health and well-being. Targeted health education in communities can bring positive behavioural change among individuals against NTDs.

2.8 Healthcare Systems and NTDs

The healthcare system serves as a cornerstone of the social structure by contributing to the social welfare and resilience of communities. The accessibility and quality of healthcare services are crucial determinants of outcomes for neglected tropical diseases (NTDs) within affected communities. Accessible healthcare facilitates early detection and diagnosis of NTDs, enabling prompt treatment initiation and disease prevention. Providing affordable treatment services and implementing preventive measures such as mass drug administration (MDA), vector control, vaccination programs and health education initiatives are essential for controlling NTD transmission and reaching underserved populations.

India faces significant challenges in delivering easily accessible healthcare to all its citizens, mainly due to its vast population and diverse healthcare system (Chawla, 2023). The accessibility issues are mainly influenced by several reasons, including vast regional inequalities, socioeconomic circumstances, infrastructure constraints and cultural diversities (Rao et al., 2011). While significant efforts have been made in recent years to enhance healthcare accessibility in the country, challenges persist, particularly in rural and economically underdeveloped regions (Panagariya, 2014).

As a country with a high NTD burden, India has implemented significant policies and programs like the National Centre for Vector Borne Disease Control (NCVBDC) and the National Leprosy Eradication Programme to control major NTDs in the country. In order to eliminate LF, the country implements an annual mass drug administration (MDA) and morbidity management among lymphedema patients. Since 2015, India has conducted the world's largest deworming initiative in schools, targeting soil-transmitted helminths (STH) in approximately 250 million children (Ajjampur et al., 2021). However, challenges such as poor community participation, systemic mistrust issues and inadequate financing continue to delay the achievement of elimination targets (Chandra et al., 2023). Despite these challenges, there have been notable successes in NTD control efforts, including reductions in kala-azar and leprosy cases in the country. Investing in healthcare infrastructure, strengthening health systems, promoting multi-sectoral collaboration and empowering communities are essential strategies for improving healthcare accessibility and achieving health equity for all to control NTDs.

2.9 Conclusion

This chapter examined the intricate interplay between NTDs and the social dimensions prevalent in India, shedding light on the significant impact of poverty, housing, sanitation, occupation, education, social identity, culture, individual behaviours and healthcare system-related factors on the prevalence, transmission and management of NTDs. It also discussed how marginalised communities in impoverished areas in the country, often trapped in a cycle of poverty and illness, bear the disproportionate burden of NTDs due to their socio-economic vulnerabilities. Through the analysis of existing literature, it becomes evident that addressing the root causes of poverty and social inequality is fundamental to breaking disease transmission in India. Moreover, holistic interventions not only focus on medical treatments but also consider social factors, with social work emerging as an important discipline playing a key role in this effort.

References

Aagaard-Hansen, J., & Chaignat, C. L. (2010). Neglected tropical diseases: Equity and social determinants. *Equity, Social Determinants and Public Health Programmes, 135*(1), 303.

Ajjampur, S. S. R., Kaliappan, S. P., Halliday, K. E., Palanisamy, G., Farzana, J., Manuel, M., Abraham, D., Laxmanan, S., Aruldas, K., Rose, A., Kennedy, D. S., Oswald, W. E., Pullan, R. L., Galagan, S. R., Ásbjörnsdóttir, K., Anderson, R. M., Muliyil, J., Sarkar, R., Kang, G., & Walson, J. L. (2021). Epidemiology of soil transmitted helminths and risk analysis of hookworm infections in the community: Results from the DeWorm3 trial in southern India. *PLoS Neglected Tropical Diseases, 15*(4), e0009338. https://doi.org/10.1371/journal.pntd.0009338

Alam, M., Yunus, M., Kalam, A., & Khan, A. (1998). Study of socio-economic factors in relation to leprosy. *Indian Journal of Community Medicine, 23*(2), 77–80.

Baru, R., Acharya, A., Acharya, S., Kumar, A. S., & Nagaraj, K. (2010). Inequities in access to health services in India: Caste, class and region. *Economic and Political Weekly, 45*, 49–58.

Behera, P., Munshi, H., Kalkonde, Y., Deshmukh, M., & Bang, A. (2021). Control of scabies in a tribal community using mass screening and treatment with oral ivermectin -a cluster randomized controlled trial in Gadchiroli, India. *PLoS Neglected Tropical Diseases, 15*(4), e0009330. https://doi.org/10.1371/journal.pntd.0009330

Bern, C., Courtenay, O., & Alvar, J. (2010). Of cattle, sand flies and men: A systematic review of risk factor analyses for south Asian visceral leishmaniasis and implications for elimination. *PLoS Neglected Tropical Diseases, 4*(2), e599. https://doi.org/10.1371/journal.pntd.0000599

Bhagat, R. B. (2018). *Urbanization in India: Trend, pattern and policy issues*. International Institute for Population Sciences.

Bhunia, G. S., Chatterjee, N., Kumar, V., Siddiqui, N. A., Mandal, R., Das, P., & Kesari, S. (2012). Delimitation of kala-azar risk areas in the district of Vaishali in Bihar (India) using a geo-environmental approach. *Memorias do Instituto Oswaldo Cruz, 107*(5), 609–620.

Bhutta, Z. A., Sommerfeld, J., Lassi, Z. S., Salam, R. A., & Das, J. K. (2014). Global burden, distribution, and interventions for infectious diseases of poverty. *Infectious Diseases of Poverty, 3*(21), 1–7.

Campbell-Lendrum, D., Manga, L., Bagayoko, M., & Sommerfeld, J. (2015). Climate change and vector-borne diseases: What are the implications for public health research and policy? *Philosophical transactions of the Royal Society of London. Series B, Biological Sciences, 370*(1665), 20130552. https://doi.org/10.1098/rstb.2013.0552

Chandra, A., Sreeganga, S. D., Rath, N., & Ramaprasad, A. (2023). Healthcare policies to eliminate neglected tropical diseases (NTDs) in India: A roadmap. *International Journal of Environmental Research and Public Health, 20*(19), 6842. https://doi.org/10.3390/ijerph20196842

Chandramouli, C. (2011). *Housing stock, amenities and assets in slums – Census 2011*. Registrar General & Census Commissioner of India. http://censusindia.gov.in/2011-Documents/On_Slums-2011Final.ppt

Chawla, N. S. (2023). Unveiling the ABCs: Identifying India's healthcare service gaps. *Cureus, 15*(7), e42398. https://doi.org/10.7759/cureus.42398

Dasgupta, U., Mani, S., Sharma, S., & Singhal, S. (2023). Social identity, behavior, and personality: Evidence from India. *The Journal of Development Studies, 59*(4), 472–489.

Datta, J., Bhattacharya, T., Chakraborty, S., Ahmed, S. K. S., Patra, A. C., Roy, S., Sarkar, A. P., & Das, N. K. (2022). Perception of leprosy patients towards the disease in a tertiary Care Hospital of High Prevalent District in West Bengal, India: A qualitative study. *Indian Journal of Dermatology, 67*(2), 206. https://doi.org/10.4103/ijd.ijd_1151_20

Erlanger, T. E., Keiser, J., Caldas De Castro, M., Bos, R., Singer, B. H., Tanner, M., & Utzinger, J. (2005). Effect of water resource development and management on lymphatic filariasis, and estimates of populations at risk. *The American Journal of Tropical Medicine and Hygiene, 73*(3), 523–533.

Faust, C. L., McCallum, H. I., Bloomfield, L. S., Gottdenker, N. L., Gillespie, T. R., Torney, C. J., et al. (2018). Pathogen spillover during land conversion. *Ecology Letters, 21*(4), 471–483.

Galgamuwa, L. S., Iddawela, D., & Dharmaratne, S. D. (2018). Prevalence and intensity of Ascaris lumbricoides infections in relation to undernutrition among children in a tea plantation community, Sri Lanka: a cross-sectional study. *BMC Pediatrics, 18*(1), 13. https://doi.org/10.1186/s12887-018-0984-3

Gang, I. N., Sen, K., & Yun, M. S. (2017). Is caste destiny? Occupational diversification among dalits in rural India. *The European Journal of Development Research, 29*, 476–492.

Garsed, C., & Waite, R. (2015). *The importance of water, sanitation and hygiene for lymphatic filariasis and leprosy care and inclusion* (Briefing note). Leprosy Mission England & Wales and Water Aid UK. Available at: https://leprosymission.contentfiles.net/media/documents/WASH_in_LF_and_leprosy_self-care_briefing_note_2.pdf. Accessed Dec 2023.

Government of India. (2019). *Drinking water, sanitation, hygiene and housing condition in India-NSS 76th round*. Available at: chrome-extension://efaidnbmnnnibpcajpcglclefindmkaj/https://www.mospi.gov.in/sites/default/files/publication_reports/Report_584_final_0.pdf

Guha, U., Chatterjee, M., Sardar, A. A., Jana, K., Saha, P., Maji, A. K., & Guha, S. K. (2020). Assessment of knowledge, attitudes, and practices about visceral Leishmaniasis in endemic areas of Malda District, West Bengal, India. *The American Journal of Tropical Medicine and Hygiene, 104*(2), 646–652.

Hotez, P. J. (2017). Global urbanization and the neglected tropical diseases. *PLoS Neglected Tropical Diseases, 11*(2), e0005308. https://doi.org/10.1371/journal.pntd.0005308

Hotez, P. J., Alvarado, M., Basáñez, M. G., Bolliger, I., Bourne, R., Boussinesq, M., et al. (2014). The global burden of disease study 2010: Interpretation and implications for the neglected tropical diseases. *PLoS Neglected Tropical Diseases, 8*(7). https://doi.org/10.1371/journal.pntd.0002865

Houweling, T. A., Karim-Kos, H. E., Kulik, M. C., Stolk, W. A., Haagsma, J. A., Lenk, E. J., Richardus, J. H., & de Vlas, S. J. (2016). Socioeconomic inequalities in neglected tropical diseases: A systematic review. *PLoS Neglected Tropical Diseases, 10*(5), e0004546. https://doi.org/10.1371/journal.pntd.0004546

ILO. (2021). Inequalities and the World of Work, Report IV. International Labour Conference, 109th session, 2021. Available at: wcms_792123%20(1).pdf.

Jacob, J. T., & Franco-Paredes, C. (2008). The stigmatization of leprosy in India and its impact on future approaches to elimination and control. *PLoS Neglected Tropical Diseases, 2*(1), e113. https://doi.org/10.1371/journal.pntd.0000113

Kolimenakis, A., Heinz, S., Wilson, M. L., Winkler, V., Yakob, L., Michaelakis, A., Papachristos, D., Richardson, C., & Horstick, O. (2021). The role of urbanisation in the spread of Aedes mosquitoes and the diseases they transmit-A systematic review. *PLoS Neglected Tropical Diseases, 15*(9), e0009631. https://doi.org/10.1371/journal.pntd.0009631

Kumar, C. J., Baboo, C. A., Krishnan, B. U., Kumar, A., Joy, S., Jose, T., et al. (2007). The socio-economic impact of the chikungunya viral epidemic in India. *Open Medicine, 1*(3), 150–152.

Magalhães, A. R., Codeço, C. T., Svenning, J. C., Escobar, L. E., Van de Vuurst, P., & Gonçalves-Souza, T. (2023). Neglected tropical diseases risk correlates with poverty and early ecosystem destruction. *Infectious Diseases of Poverty, 12*(1), 32.

Mandal, N. K., & Saha, G. (2015). A qualitative assessment of current perception of different social groups about leprosy in High & low Prevalent Districts of West Bengal. *Journal of Comprehensive Health, 3*(2), 23–32.

Modi, A., Vaishnav, K. G., Kothiya, K., & Alexander, N. (2021). Lymphatic filariasis elimination endgame in an urban Indian setting: The roles of surveillance and residual microfilaremia after mass drug administration. *Infectious Diseases of Poverty, 10*(1), 73. https://doi.org/10.1186/s40249-021-00856-x

Murhekar, M. V., Kamaraj, P., Kumar, M. S., Khan, S. A., Allam, R. R., Barde, P., et al. (2019). Burden of dengue infection in India, 2017: A cross-sectional population based serosurvey. *The Lancet Global Health, 7*(8), 1065–1073.

Mutheneni, S. R., Upadhyayula, S. M., Kumaraswamy, S., Kadiri, M. R., & Nagalla, B. (2016). Influence of socioeconomic aspects on lymphatic filariasis: A case-control study in Andhra Pradesh, India. *Journal of Vector Borne Diseases, 53*(3), 272–278.

Nair, P. A., Vora, R. V., Jivani, N. B., & Gandhi, S. S. (2016). A study of clinical profile and quality of life in patients with scabies at a rural tertiary care centre. *Journal of Clinical and Diagnostic Research: JCDR, 10*(10), 1–5.

Nayak, R., Panda, M., Padhy, S., & Mishra, K. G. (2021). Paradigm shift in socio-demographic profile of dengue infection: A hospital based cross-sectional study. *Journal of Family Medicine and Primary Care, 10*(6), 2405–2410.

Nguela, R. L., Bigoga, J. D., Armel, T. N., Esther, T., Line, D., Boris, N. A., et al. (2020). The effect of improved housing on indoor mosquito density and exposure to malaria in the rural community of Minkoameyos, Centre region of Cameroon. *Malaria Journal, 19*(1), 1–16.

Panagariya, A. (2014). The challenges and innovative solutions to rural health dilemma. *Annals of Neurosciences, 21*(4), 125–127.

Paulson, W., Kodali, N. K., Balasubramani, K., et al. (2022). Social and housing indicators of dengue and chikungunya in Indian adults aged 45 and above: Analysis of a nationally representative survey (2017–18). *Archives of Public Health, 80*, 125. https://doi.org/10.1186/s13690-022-00868-5

Perry, D., Dixon, K., Garlapati, R., Gendernalik, A., Poché, D., & Poché, R. (2013a). Visceral leishmaniasis prevalence and associated risk factors in the saran district of Bihar, India, from 2009 to July of 2011. *The American Journal of Tropical Medicine and Hygiene, 88*(4), 778–784.

Perry, D., Dixon, K., Garlapati, R., Gendernalik, A., Poché, D., & Poché, R. (2013b). Visceral leishmaniasis prevalence and associated risk factors in the saran district of Bihar, India, from 2009 to July of 2011. *American Journal of Tropical Medicine and Hygiene, 88*(4), 778–784.

Pescarini, J. M., Strina, A., Nery, J. S., Skalinski, L. M., Andrade, K. V. F., Penna, M. L. F., Brickley, E. B., Rodrigues, L. C., Barreto, M. L., & Penna, G. O. (2018). Socioeconomic risk markers of leprosy in high-burden countries: A systematic review and meta-analysis. *PLoS Neglected Tropical Diseases, 12*(7), e0006622. https://doi.org/10.1371/journal.pntd.0006622

Prist, P. R., Uriarte, M., Tambosi, L. R., Prado, A., Pardini, R., Andrea, D., & P. S., & Metzger, J. P. (2016). Landscape, environmental and social predictors of hantavirus risk in São Paulo, Brazil. *PLoS One, 11*(10), e0163459. https://doi.org/10.1371/journal.pone.0163459

Priyamvada, K., Bindroo, J., Sharma, M. P., Chapman, L. A. C., Dubey, P., Mahapatra, T., Hightower, A. W., Bern, C., & Srikantiah, S. (2021). Visceral leishmaniasis outbreaks in Bihar: Community-level investigations in the context of elimination of kala-azar as a public health problem. *Parasites & Vectors, 14*(1), 52. https://doi.org/10.1186/s13071-020-04551-y

Raghavendra, R. H. (2020). Literacy and health status of scheduled castes in India. *Contemporary Voice of Dalit, 12*(1), 97–110.

Rao, M., Rao, K. D., Kumar, A. S., Chatterjee, M., & Sundararaman, T. (2011). Human resources for health in India. *The Lancet, 377*(9765), 587–598.

Salam, N., & Azam, S. (2017). Prevalence and distribution of soil-transmitted helminth infections in India. *BMC Public Health, 17*(1), 1–12.

Saleem, M., Burdett, T., & Heaslip, V. (2019). Health and social impacts of open defecation on women: A systematic review. *BMC Public Health, 19*(1), 1–12.

Sen, A. (1983). Poor, relatively speaking. *Oxford Economic Papers, 35*(2), 153–169.

Stephen, T., Selvaraj, I., & Parameswari, P. J. (2014). Assessment of knowledge, attitude and practice about leprosy among patients and their families in a rural community in Tamil Nadu. *Indian Journal of Leprosy, 86*(1), 7–14.

Sundar, S., Singh, O. P., & Chakravarty, J. (2018). Visceral leishmaniasis elimination targets in India, strategies for preventing resurgence. *Expert Review of Anti-Infective Therapy, 16*(11), 805–812.

Swain, S., Bhatt, M., Biswal, D., Pati, S., & Magalhaes, R. J. S. (2020). Risk factors for dengue outbreaks in Odisha, India: A case-control study. *Journal of Infection and Public Health, 13*(4), 625–631.

Swaminathan, S., Perumal, V., Adinarayanan, S., Kaliannagounder, K., Rengachari, R., & Purushothaman, J. (2012). Epidemiological assessment of eight rounds of mass drug administration for lymphatic filariasis in India: Implications for monitoring and evaluation. *PLoS Neglected Tropical Diseases, 6*(11), e1926. https://doi.org/10.1371/journal.pntd.0001926

Telle, O., Vaguet, A., Yadav, N. K., Lefebvre, B., Daudé, E., Paul, R. E., et al. (2016). The spread of dengue in an endemic urban milieu–the case of Delhi, India. *PLoS One, 11*(3), e0152847. https://doi.org/10.1371/journal.pone.0152847

Traub, R. J., Robertson, I. D., Irwin, P., Mencke, N., & Andrew Thompson, R. C. (2004). The prevalence, intensities and risk factors associated with geohelminth infection in tea-growing communities of Assam, India. *Tropical Medicine & International Health, 9*(6), 688–701.

Tripathi, B., Roy, N., & Dhingra, N. (2022). Introduction of triple-drug therapy for accelerating lymphatic filariasis elimination in India: lessons learned. *The American Journal of Tropical Medicine and Hygiene, 106*(5 Suppl), 29.

Trivedi, S., & Chakravarty, A. (2022). Neurological complications of dengue fever. *Current Neurology and Neuroscience Reports, 22*(8), 515–529.

Tullu, M. S., & Karande, S. (2009). Leptospirosis in children: A review for family physicians. *Indian Journal of Medical Sciences, 63*(8), 368–378.

UNESCO. (2019). *Global education monitoring report*. Available at: https://www.unesco.org/gem-report/en/2019-gender-report

United Nations, Department of Economic and Social Affairs. (2018). *Revision of World urbanization prospects*. Available at: https://www.un.org/en/desa/2018-revision-world-urbanization-prospects#:~:text=The%20urban%20population%20of%20the,and%20Africa%20with%2013%25%20each

Upadhyayula, S. M., Mutheneni, S. R., Kadiri, M. R., Kumaraswamy, S., & Nagalla, B. (2012). A cohort study of lymphatic filariasis on socio economic conditions in Andhra Pradesh, India. *PLoS One, 7*(3), e33779. https://doi.org/10.1371/journal.pone.0033779

Wani, S. A., & Ahmad, F. (2009). Intestinal helminths and associated risk factors in children of district Pulwama, Kashmir, India. *Indian Journal of Medical Microbiology, 27*(1), 81–82.

Williams, T., Karim, M. J., Uddin, S., Jahan, S., Asm, S. M., Forbes, S. P., et al. (2023). Socio-economic and environmental factors associated with high lymphatic filariasis morbidity prevalence distribution in Bangladesh. *PLoS Neglected Tropical Diseases, 17*(7), e0011457. https://doi.org/10.1371/journal.pntd.0011457

World Health Organization. (2017). *Integrating neglected tropical diseases into global health and development: Fourth WHO report on neglected tropical diseases*. World Health Organization. Available at: http://apps.who.int/iris/bitstream/10665/255011/1/9789241565448-eng.pdf

World Health Organization. (2024). *Leishmaniasis*. Available at: https://www.who.int/india/health-topics/leishmaniasis

Chapter 3
Social Work for the Control and Elimination of Neglected Tropical Diseases

3.1 Introduction

This chapter is an exploration of the vital role that social work plays in addressing neglected tropical diseases (NTDs). It delves into various aspects, ranging from the limitations of the medical model to the integration of community and medical social work practices. This chapter emphasises principles, strategies and ethical considerations while also highlighting the role of social workers in multi-disciplinary teams and the significance of cultural competence and social work research for addressing NTDs. In essence, this chapter throws light on the role of social workers as important team members in the multidisciplinary teams working on the control and elimination of NTDs and argues for the importance of including social work as an essential component in the global NTD control and prevention programmes.

3.2 Positioning Social Work as a Key Profession for Eliminating NTDs

Ever since the WHO's increased emphasis on the need for the elimination of NTDs, global efforts have been put into the elimination of NTDs, and NTDs have become a major public health subject matter. In the global battle against NTDs, various international organisations, including the WHO and the US Centers for Disease Control and Prevention (CDC), have developed specific strategic interventions for preventing, controlling and eliminating these diseases (WHO, 2010; CDC, 2023). Their strategies typically involve innovative disease management, preventive chemotherapy, vector control, veterinary public health, and the provision of safe water, sanitation and hygiene in endemic settings. Additionally, the CDC recommends

© The Author(s), under exclusive license to Springer Nature Switzerland AG 2024
M. Jabir, A. C. Choolayil, *Social Work with Populations Vulnerable to Neglected Tropical Diseases*, SpringerBriefs in Social Work,
https://doi.org/10.1007/978-3-031-68997-0_3

policy development, research, monitoring and capacity building. Notably, the WHO's recent strategic framework for skin-related NTDs emphasised the need for social mobilisation, active case detection, clinical and laboratory diagnosis, rehabilitation, self-care, stigma reduction, inclusion, human rights and support systems (WHO, 2021).

Current frameworks for NTD control underscore the importance of collaborative effort from professionals with diverse skills and knowledge for enhanced programme outcomes. Despite social workers increasingly playing critical roles in global health by providing behavioural health interventions, care coordination, programme planning, resource mobilisation, and research for illness prevention and health promotion, none of these frameworks has a clear-cut role for social workers in NTD interventions. In contrast, most of these frameworks primarily prioritise medical and allied health professionals in NTD programmes. However, NTD control and elimination essentially involve roles that align with the profession's philosophy, even though traditional health social work literature rarely discusses NTDs, primarily because these diseases are prevalent in tropical countries or resource-limited countries, where social work is still evolving. Most of the recorded literature on the origins and development of professional social work is in Europe and the United States, where NTDs are less prevalent, and the early literature on social work has little to no reference to social work for NTDs. Even after the evolution of social work as a recognised profession associated with public health, the nature and role of social work for NTDs remained ambiguous and unrecorded due to the fact that global social work literature largely revolved around the practices and advancements in the West. NTDs were and are prevalent among African and Southeast Asian countries, where the social work profession is still evolving and only gradually being recognised as a key profession (Baikady et al., 2021; Chitereka, 2009). Also, the limited global attention to NTDs until the early 2000s meant that the social work profession had very little recorded history of working for the cause of preventing and eliminating NTDs until recently.

Social workers have been engaging in NTD programmes in the Asian and African contexts but with limited demarcated roles. Due to these limited demarcated roles, health social workers are seldom considered essential professionals in the programmes that target the control and elimination of NTDs. In the cases where social workers are part of the NTD control and prevention programme, the roles are not well defined, and the unique impact of social work is not recorded. This is mostly because the NTD programmes often involve multidisciplinary teams where the role and scope of social work are not well acknowledged. These aspects create a gap in the traditional social work literature on what constitutes health social work for NTDs. This leads to the question of whether such a body of literature is essential or rather whether a generic literature of health social work can address the components of social work practice associated with NTDs.

3.3 Towards a Social Work Model for Working with NTDs

Given the ambiguity of the nature of social work with NTDs and the lack of recorded literature, despite social workers constantly engaging in NTD programmes, it is essential that the basics of social work for NTDs be laid down from existing evidence—both theoretical and practical. The aim is to underscore the relevance of social work discipline in eliminating NTDs by highlighting the strengths of this profession that can contribute to achieving the target of NTD elimination. The limited recognition of social work with NTDs can primarily be due to the tendency in public health research to label all social disciplines as homogenous, failing to recognise the strengths and uniqueness of multiple social sciences disciplines (Allotey et al., 2010). This generalisation of the social sciences disciplines under an umbrella in the public health sector has adversely affected social science disciplines working on public health issues, including social work. In order to demarcate the role and relevance of social work discipline in controlling and eliminating NTDs, the nature and salient features of social work that make it a relevant discipline in the subject matter are to be laid down. Social work, undoubtedly, occupies a pivotal role in the global health landscape.

We propose a new social work model that integrates social workers into key positions within NTD control programmes (Fig. 3.1). The purpose of this model is to address the ambiguity surrounding the role of social work in combating NTDs and underscore the relevance of the social work discipline in eliminating NTDs by highlighting its strengths and unique contributions. The model encompasses the following six domains: epidemiology; vector control; clinical and case management;

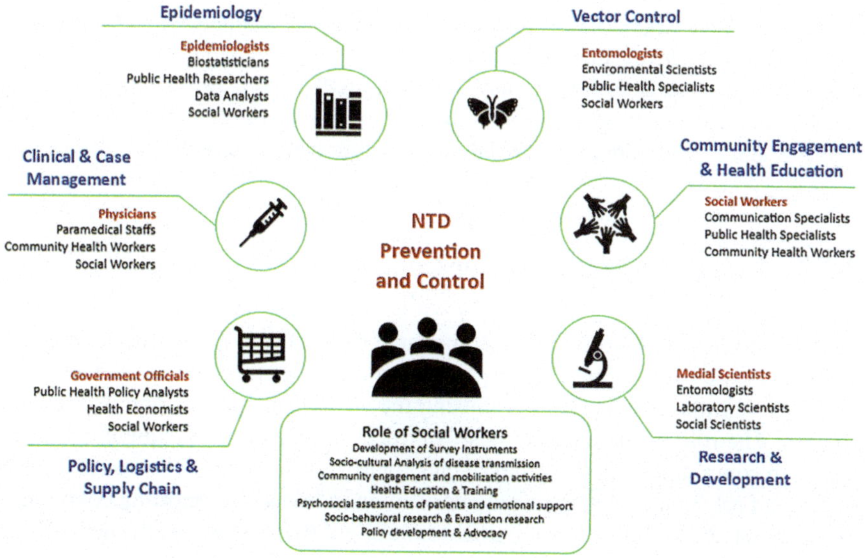

Fig. 3.1 Social workers in NTD control

community engagement and health education; research and development; and policy and logistics (including supply chain management). By emphasising the socio-economic and cultural aspects of NTDs, this model aims to demonstrate the vital role of social workers in NTD programmes.

3.3.1 Role of Social Workers in Epidemiological Analysis of NTDs

Epidemiology serves as an important cross-cutting activity in any NTD control programme that aims to understand the prevalence, distribution and dynamics of the diseases in the given population, with a specific focus on their prevention. This plays a crucial role in informing evidence-based decision-making and designing targeted interventions. The epidemiology team generally include health professionals, biostatisticians, public health scientists, data analysts and social scientists. The social scientists play a vital role in this team by enhancing the team's understanding of the broader contextual factors that influence disease transmission, including the social determinants that shape health outcomes.

The success of any NTD programme starts with the programme being culturally sensitive and socially relevant. Although the medical field recognises the importance of comprehending and being mindful of the socio-cultural setting in which a health intervention is implemented, it lacks the depth and breadth of understanding these subtleties as social sciences disciplines do. The social work profession, in particular, is not just an academic discipline but a practice-based profession that works with people based on its principle of social justice, emphasising respect for diversity (IFSW, 2018). Social workers are trained professionals who can grasp the socio-cultural nuances that influence health-seeking behaviours and impact the effectiveness of interventions. They can support the team in developing survey instruments and ensuring the team's analyses and interventions are scientifically rigorous and considerate of the social fabric within which these diseases manifest.

3.3.2 Social Workers in Vector Control

Vector control is another important component in NTD control that focuses on controlling diseases transmitting vectors, such as mosquitoes, sandflies, ticks and mites. This intervention is critical in minimising the vector's abundance and its breeding sources. The role of the entomologist is critical in this group in studying vectors, their behaviour and their surveillance and control activities. Social workers have a significant role in the vector control intervention in terms of supporting community engagement and mobilisation activities, thereby enhancing the effectiveness of vector control strategies. They can serve as liaisons between the vector control team and local communities affected by NTD. Additionally, they can engage in community assessments to understand the sociocultural dynamics and perceptions related to the adoption of vector control measures, thereby designing and implementing tailored health education campaigns that focus on behavioural change and sustainable practices that align with vector control goals.

3.3.3 *Integrating Social Work into Clinical and Case Management of NTD Patients*

Clinical and case management is another core strategic component in the framework that focuses on providing medical care, treatment, and psychosocial support to patients affected by NTDs. This intervention ensures timely and effective service delivery for improved health outcomes. In this activity, the role of physicians and other health professionals is critical. The social worker can work in a supportive role in addressing the psychosocial aspects of patients by conducting psychosocial assessments to identify their unique needs. Additionally, they can offer counselling and emotional support to the patients to help individuals cope with the challenges associated with their conditions. They can collaborate closely with physicians to develop holistic care plans that encompass not only medical treatments but also psychosocial and community-based support. Finally, their contribution towards reducing the social stigma associated with NTDs, promoting inclusivity, and fostering community understanding and patient follow-up in treatment is invaluable.

3.3.4 *Empowering Communities: Social Worker's Role in Community Engagement and Health Education for NTD Control*

Like any other disease, community engagement and health education emerge as an indispensable element in the holistic framework to prevent and control NTD in India. Community engagement is 'a process of developing relationships that enable stakeholders to work together to address health-related issues and promote well-being to achieve positive health impact and outcomes' (WHO, 2020a, b. Community engagement will help create trust, mobilise extra resources in resource-constrained settings and facilitate a sustainable collaborating atmosphere to achieve better health outcomes (Attree et al., 2011; Popay et al., 2007). WHO (2020a, b) stresses that health interventions should be community-oriented, community-based and community-owned for better health promotion and outcomes. The national programmes to combat NTDs in India, such as the National Centre for Vector Borne Diseases Control (NCVBDC), have also emphasised that effective community engagement is needed along with epidemiological surveillance and vector control for the prevention and control of NTDs like dengue and filariasis.

In the Indian context, community engagement stands as a linchpin in the prevention of neglected tropical diseases (NTDs). The diverse and vast landscape of India, coupled with varying socioeconomic and cultural factors, necessitates a localised and community-driven approach to effectively combat NTDs such as dengue, filariasis, Zika, chikungunya and other NTDs. By actively involving communities, public health initiatives gain access to invaluable local knowledge, allowing for the identification of breeding sites, understanding disease patterns and tailoring interventions accordingly. Additionally, community engagement fosters a sense of ownership and responsibility among individuals, promoting sustained behavioural changes crucial for vector control and disease prevention.

The community engagement and health education intervention can be delivered by a team comprising social workers, health educators and communication experts. Social workers can play a lead role, leveraging their expertise in assessing community needs, concerns and cultural contexts. Interventions and programmes addressing NTDs are community-based interventions like MDA and vector management strategies. Often, the success and failure of such programmes depend on the participation of the community. While multiple disciplines engage in community mobilisation and organisation efforts, the social work profession specialises in engaging communities and empowering them through participatory approaches (Adams, 2017). Social work professionals possess the expertise to elicit community engagement in health programmes, which is one of the key factors that determine the success of most NTD programmes. Rooted in the principles of community organisation, particularly the principles of democratic functioning, flexible organisation and cultural orientation (Gangrade, 1971; Harper & Dunham, 1959; Ross, 1967), trained social worker professionals can ensure that the community participates, engages and owns the health programmes that are targeted for NTD elimination. What makes the social work profession different from other professions in this regard is that the core social work practice with the community is essentially participatory and, hence, professional social workers can integrate themselves into the team of NTD programmes with ease.

In the context of NTDs, where cultural beliefs, social practices and community dynamics are integral, social workers can serve as cultural brokers, facilitating effective communication between health providers and communities. This understanding is essential for tailoring interventions to the unique needs and perspectives of the community. The unique positioning of social, both as an academic discipline and a practice-based profession, makes it ideal for engaging in culturally sensitive and socially relevant models for addressing NTDs. Moreover, community networks and ties are important in eliminating health system distrust, which is a major reason for non-adherence to preventive treatments like MDA and vaccination (Adams et al., 2018). Community social work, by virtue of its very foundational principles, engages in building connection and trust with community structures like institutions, local leaders and community-based organisations to strengthen social ties. This practice is unique to the social work profession, where the community can be the agent of change, the target of change or the context for change (Coulton, 2005). In the context of NTDs, the interventions need to consider the fact that elimination or control is feasible only through community participation. Non-adherence by the community could be due to socio-economic factors, religious factors, cultural factors and health system distrust. The success of the intervention programmes, in such scenarios, solely relies on the effectiveness of garnering community support effectively. Community social work specialises in acquiring community trust and cooperation by networking with the community structures.

Furthermore, health education and promotion are core strategies that support community engagement in NTD control. As many of these diseases are preventable, better health promotion interventions play a significant role in NTD control and prevention. Studies have found that health education is crucial in NTD prevention, and it can significantly contribute to better outcomes in a shorter timeframe and at a lower cost (Chandra et al., 2023; Garapati et al., 2018). Social workers could support in designing and implementing health education campaigns that not only disseminate information about NTDs but also address the underlying social, economic and cultural factors that may impact their health outcomes. Through their role as cultural competence specialists, social workers ensure that interventions are respectful of diverse cultural norms, fostering a sense of trust and understanding within the community. They can be involved in regular health education campaigns to create a sense of ownership and responsiveness regarding their health among community members. They can also contribute to the training of community health workers in health education at the grassroots level. In addition, they can mobilise communities for active participation in NTD prevention efforts and fostering sustainable health practices.

3.3.5 Integrating Social Work Research in NTD Control

The research and development component in this model supports all other activities in terms of advancing scientific knowledge; developing new interventions; and improving diagnostics, drugs and vaccines for NTD control. In this process, the medical researchers, clinicians, laboratory scientists and drug and vaccine researchers play an important role. While medical scientists and other researchers develop drugs and vaccines and validate them in real-life situations, social scientists can play integral roles in enriching the research process with a human-centric and community-focused approach. Their expertise facilitates the incorporation of local insights into research design. By employing qualitative research methods, they can provide valuable insights into social and behavioural factors influencing NTDs, conducting interviews, focus groups and observational studies. Additionally, they act as advocates for ethical considerations, addressing issues related to informed consent, privacy and confidentiality. Their involvement can ensure that research efforts are not only scientifically rigorous but also socially responsible, ethically sound and rooted in the lived experiences of those affected by NTDs.

3.3.6 *Role of Social Workers in Policy Advocacy and Logistics Management*

The model suggests policy, logistics and supply chain components that focus on advocating for policies, coordinating logistics, and ensuring the efficient procurement, storage and distribution of resources to support NTD control. The role of public health policy analysts and the respective state and union governments is crucial in this intervention. Social workers can contribute insights into the social determinants of health and equity in policy formulation and implementation. They can be involved in community impact assessments to gauge the potential effects of policies on different populations, particularly those in underserved communities. Additionally, their engagement extends to facilitating community involvement in policy development, collaborating with stakeholders and providing psychosocial support during logistics and supply chain management. By advocating for resource allocation and supporting crisis intervention strategies, social workers can contribute not only to the effective implementation of policies but also to the overall resilience and well-being of communities affected by NTDs.

Overall, as NTDs are a group of infectious diseases that disproportionately affect impoverished communities, as discussed in the previous chapter, social workers, with their unique skill set and commitment to social justice, are instrumental in creating holistic strategies and interventions to address the diseases. While the list of unique sets of roles that social workers can offer to NTD programmes mentioned above is not comprehensive, it is an attempt to lay down how the social work profession can be pivotal in the programmes targeting NTDs. The aim is not to comprehensively list all the roles that social workers can perform in NTD programmes but to highlight how social workers can contribute to the NTD programme and the team in unique ways or through better methods that other professions cannot. This is done in view of the scarcity of literature that lays down the unique set of roles that social workers have in NTD control and prevention. With this unique set of skills, social workers can contribute to the multidisciplinary teams that work towards the control and elimination of NTDs.

3.4 Integrating Community and Clinical Models for NTD Social Work

The social work profession, from its nascent phase, emphasised its role in the public health domain through clinical social work and community social work, known as the 'dual heartbeat' of social work (Ruth & Marshall, 2017). Though working towards the same cause, grounded on the principle of social justice, these methods are often demarcated and reserved for specific settings. Often, the idea of health social work is synonymous with hospital social work and thereby labelled to be pertaining to clinical social work. While health social work essentially involves clinical components and health social workers engage in healthcare settings predominantly, the role of health social work in community settings is of equal importance. While clinical social work addresses the social and psychological needs of individuals and families, community social work engages in structural reforms aimed at improving community well-being (Ruth & Marshall, 2017). However, NTDs constitute a case where health social workers have to integrate community and clinical social work components to successfully address the question of behavioural change and structural modifications necessary to address the overlapping behavioural and structural determinants of health.

NTDs constitute a case of intersection of personal and structural components, making individuals vulnerable to ill health. Traditionally, health social work models are often constrained to medical models with a focus on individual behaviour as the causative factor for poor health outcomes (Blue et al., 2016). NTDs essentially involve behavioural elements and structural elements in such a way that certain behavioural elements are sometimes induced by structural deficits. Hence, in order to address the risk of NTDs, addressing the structural and the behavioural components is equally important. This demand for structural and behavioural intervention requires that any social work intervention aimed at facilitating the control and prevention of NTDs integrates both clinical social work methods and community social work methods effectively. The clinical models, mostly casework, shall be helpful in targeting the persuasion of power centres, promoting preventive measures and morbidity management, and targeting power centres and stakeholders of critical importance. The community model, on the other hand, can work with larger groups targeting a larger level of impact, such as enabling communities to engage in and own vector control programmes, promoting mass drug administration (MDA) and health education, etc. The community model shall be helpful in addressing the macro aspects of NTDs, and the clinical model shall be helpful in addressing the micro aspects of NTDs. This combination of the clinical and the community model is an essential component for working with NTDs. However, recognising social work as a relevant profession in addressing the problem of NTDs is still not a subject matter adequately discussed and well defined in the literature.

3.5 Ethical Standards in Working with Communities Vulnerable to NTDs

Ethical principles act as a guiding moral compass for social workers, directing their actions and decisions by the fundamental values of the profession. Several international social work organisations attempted to formulate general ethical principles that social workers are obligated to adhere to regardless of their field of practice. Notably, the ethical principles established by the National Association of Social Workers (NASW), USA, in 1960 have gained widespread acceptance among social work organisations worldwide (Reamer, 2006). These standards encompass ethical obligations towards clients, colleagues, practice settings, the profession and society at large. They are rooted in core values such as social justice, the inherent dignity and worth of individuals, the significance of human relationships, integrity, and competence (NASW, 2024). In India, numerous national-level organisations have been founded to support social work professionals, and they have devised specific ethical guidelines tailored to professionals practising within the country. For example, the National Association of Professional Social Workers in India (NAPSW) has crafted ethical standards encompassing principles such as human rights and dignity, social justice, integrity, inclusivity, sustainability, service provision and interpersonal relationships (NAPSW, 2015).

Neglected tropical diseases (NTDs) are diseases of poverty, and elimination programmes are operated in a complex socio-cultural environment. NTD control programmes often require context-specific or disease-specific approaches, which present many ethical challenges (Addiss et al., 2021). Additionally, the intervention strategies differ for each NTD based on the vector species, breeding habitats, clinical manifestations and characteristics of individuals affected by the disease. For instance, the control strategy for LF and STH heavily relies on preventive chemotherapy, whereas dengue is addressed mainly through preventive methods and disease management.

Moreover, these diseases contribute to a vicious cycle of poverty, which subsequently presents neglect, deprivation, stigma and health inequity in society (Bailey et al., 2019). Some NTD programmes present particular ethical challenges as the preventive measures often involve restricting the movement of people in the affected region, leading to the loss of their livelihood and associated financial burden. Given the Indian context, these diseases are mostly affected by ethnic minorities, oppressed classes and backward communities in the deprived areas. For instance, STH is the major public health problem among many of the primitive tribes in Odisha in India. Data shows that it is prevalent among 44.6% of Bondos, 44.9% of Didayis and 41.1% of Kondha primitive tribes (ICMR, 2003). Therefore, working with these vulnerable sections requires a strong understanding of their cultural values and adherence to high ethical standards to ensure that interventions are respectful, culturally sensitive and beneficial to the community.

Below are some key ethical standards that can guide social workers in their work with communities vulnerable to NTDs:

(a) *Beneficence and Non-maleficence*: First and foremost, the sole aim of the NTD control interventions should be the well-being of affected communities. Social workers should assess the potential risks and benefits of interventions implemented. For instance, when developing strategies for controlling disease or support services in the community, social workers must ensure that the service protocols are safe for vulnerable populations, including young children, pregnant women, older adults and other groups, taking into account potential physical and emotional disturbance to them. For instance, the DA and IDA-based chemotherapy against LF is not recommended for children below 2 years, pregnant women and chronically ill individuals (WHO, 2019). In addition, the social stigma and discrimination associated with many NTDs such as LF and leprosy are prevalent in many communities across India (Kumari et al., 2010). Therefore, social workers involved in NTD control programmes are required to ensure that interventions are evidence-based, culturally appropriate, and do not cause any harm to the communities. They should ensure that the social and psychological dimensions of the diseases are addressed properly, as many of the NTDs, such as LF, create considerable social stigma among the patients.

(b) *Cultural Sensitivity*: Cultural sensitivity is essential for social workers when working with diverse communities affected by NTDs in India. They should understand and respect the cultural beliefs, values and practices of different communities, especially ethnic communities living in disease-endemic areas. This involves engaging with community leaders, acknowledging their perspectives and adapting interventions to align with cultural norms and preferences. Studies show that more than half of the patients in remote and village areas in India believe in luck and superstition concerning illness (Banerjee & Varma, 2013). Additionally, religious faith healing and traditional healing are prevalent in many parts of the country (Saha et al., 2021). Therefore, in regions where superstitions and traditional healing practices are prevalent, such as tribal and rural areas, cultural sensitivity is crucial. Social workers should collaborate with local healers and the community, incorporating indigenous knowledge about medicinal plants and local customs to ensure cultural acceptance and effectiveness of the intervention.

(c) *Competence*: Competence refers to possessing the requisite knowledge, skills and self-awareness necessary to carry out social work responsibilities effectively in a specific field. Social workers involved in tackling NTDs must possess a deep understanding of the diseases falling within this category, their causes and general methods for mitigation. Additionally, they should be well-versed in ethical principles governing their interactions with individuals, families, groups, organisations and communities affected by NTDs. Continuous professional development is crucial for social workers in the NTD domain. They must actively seek opportunities to improve their knowledge and skills, ensuring they remain abreast of emerging trends and best practices. By continuously improving their proficiency, social workers can enhance the quality and effectiveness of their interventions, thereby maximising their impact on NTD-affected populations. Furthermore, they should actively contribute to the body of knowledge within this field through research and innovative interventions. By conducting research and implementing evidence-based practices, they can contribute to the development of effective strategies for NTD prevention, treatment and management. By upholding high standards of competency, they can ensure that the services provided by the social workers are effective and aimed at the best interest of the affected population in NTDs.

(d) *Respect for Autonomy*: Like many other programmes, the social workers implementing intervention for NTDs should respect the communities' autonomy and right to self-determination. They should ensure that the community understand the purpose, risks and benefits of the intervention. This can be ensured by obtaining informed consent for participation, allowing them to make voluntary decisions. For instance, for social workers involved in any drug distribution programmes like MDA for LF, the participants should be provided with information in their local language on the potential benefits and side effects. Similarly, the treatment of children for certain NTDs, such as STH, should consider the consent of their parents to treat their children, as choking deaths were reported related to deworming medicines (WHO, 2007).

(e) *Equity and Social Justice*: Equity and social justice are key ethical elements for NTD control programmes, as these diseases predominantly affect the poor section of society. Especially in India, addressing NTDs requires a commitment to equity and social justice, particularly for marginalised communities. In many disease-endemic regions where access to healthcare is limited, social workers may advocate for equity and social justice in the provision of healthcare and resources for communities vulnerable to NTDs. This involves addressing underlying structural inequalities that contribute to health disparities. They have the responsibility to advocate for addressing social determinants of health, such as poverty education and lack of sanitation. This could involve lobbying for government initiatives to provide free or subsidised treatment for NTDs in deprived areas, ensuring all affected populations receive standard care.

(f) *Confidentiality and Privacy*: Maintaining confidentiality and privacy is a core ethical principle when working with communities affected by NTDs in India. Social workers should ensure that sensitive information shared during assessments or interventions is protected, respecting the privacy rights of individuals and families. They should ensure that data is securely stored and only accessed by authorised personnel. The ICMR national ethical guidelines for health research, 2017, have stressed the importance of maintaining confidentiality in health research and interventions (ICMR, 2017). It is the responsibility of the researcher to safeguard the entrusted information, including protecting it from unauthorised access, use, disclosure, modification, loss or theft. Social workers are often involved in community health screenings for NTDs in endemic settings. As discussed earlier, the social stigma surrounding some NTDs is significant. So, the leakage of medical information may lead to stigma and discrimination of people in the community. They should keep this confidential information to prevent discrimination and to protect an individual's privacy and dignity. It is also applicable when they are engaged in counselling or support services. Maintaining confidentiality fosters trust and facilitates the success of interventions by encouraging open communication between social workers and community members.

(g) *Collaboration and Community Engagement*: Effective NTD interventions require meaningful engagement with community members, stakeholders and other professionals, as discussed earlier. Social workers should involve community leaders and members in the planning, implementation and evaluation of interventions, ensuring that their voices are heard and their needs are addressed. Collaboration fosters empowerment, ownership and sustainability of interventions within the community. For instance, in regions affected by LF, dengue and

VL, social workers can collaborate with local leaders, self-help groups (SHGs), NGOs and healthcare providers to implement vector control measures and promote early detection and treatment of the diseases. The lack of community engagement and collaboration may lead to the poor performance of control programmes. For instance, the MDA has been administered in the LF-endemic districts in the country since 2004. However, treatment coverage and drug compliance remain sub-optimal in most of the districts, mainly attributed to poor community participation and engagement (Babu & Babu, 2014; Banerjee et al., 2019). This reminds us that NTD intervention programmes require effective community participation and collaboration.

(h) *Integrity and Transparency*: Social workers should uphold the ethical principles of integrity and transparency in their interactions with communities vulnerable to NTDs. This includes being honest about the purpose and scope of interventions, acknowledging limitations and uncertainties, and ensuring that community members have access to accurate information to make informed decisions. For instance, when conducting educational workshops on dengue prevention in urban slums, social workers are transparent about the limitations of available resources and empower community members to take proactive measures, such as eliminating breeding sites for mosquitoes and seeking prompt medical attention for symptoms.

Figure 3.2 gives an overview of ethical standards that social workers need to uphold while combating NTDs in India effectively.

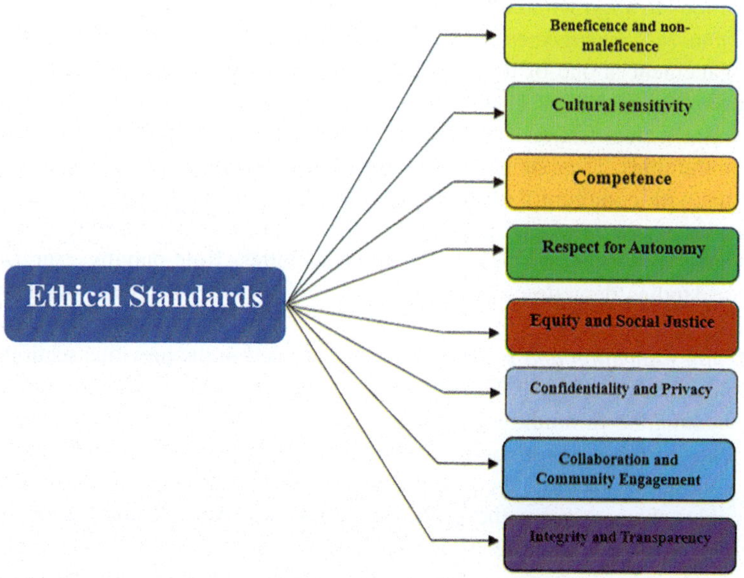

Fig. 3.2 Ethical standards for social workers in NTD control

3.6 Capacity Building for Social Workers in NTD

In the Indian context, addressing NTDs within the framework of social work education presents numerous opportunities when the graduates are equipped with the necessary knowledge and skills. Given the diverse diseases, sociocultural contexts and complex challenges associated with NTD control in the country, social workers require specific skills, knowledge and competencies to carry out their roles effectively. So, capacity building and training are essential for social workers who work for NTDs in India. Some key areas for capacity building and training include the following:

(a) *Understanding the Epidemiology of NTDs*: Social workers need a comprehensive knowledge of the various NTDs prevalent in India, including their causes, transmission methods, symptoms, treatment options and preventive measures. This will help them accurately assess the factors associated with diseases in particular contexts and address community needs, identify priority areas for intervention and effectively communicate with community members about NTD-related issues. Additionally, the knowledge of NTDs will help them to plan and implement socio-behavioural change communication and research.

(b) *Cultural Competence*: Given India's diverse cultural landscape, social workers must be trained to be sensitive regarding the beliefs, practices and customs of different communities across the country, especially the cultural practices of communities affected by NTD. Training should focus on developing cultural awareness, sensitivity to cultural taboos, superstitions, traditional healing practices, social structures, communication skills and strategies for adapting interventions to align with cultural norms and preferences.

(c) *Community Engagement and Mobilisation*: As discussed earlier, community engagement is one of the core activities for social workers involved in NTD control programmes. Therefore, they should be trained in community engagement and mobilisation techniques to facilitate the active participation of affected communities. They should learn methods and techniques for building relationships with community leaders and other stakeholders, conducting community meetings and focus group discussions, and empowering community members to take ownership of NTD prevention activities. Role-playing exercises and case studies depicting culturally sensitive scenarios can help social workers develop these skills.

(d) *Health Education and Promotion*: As mentioned in the previous sections, control and elimination of NTDs require gaining the trust of the community and educating the communities on the causes, effects and preventive strategies. The social work profession, particularly the community organisation method, helps communities identify their problems and needs through education and thus enables them to solve the problems (Baldock, 1974). Helping a community understand what leads to NTDs and how it affects their lives is elementary in bringing about change in people's perception towards the disease being addressed. The success of intervention programmes depends on the degree to which people understand these concepts, and this significantly affects their participation. Social work methods address this aspect, as the profession essentially involves engaging the community through education. Social workers play a key role in health education and promotion activities in communities aimed at raising awareness about NTDs, their symptoms, prevention and treatment. Training should equip social workers with effective communication techniques, health education materials and strategies for delivering culturally appropriate health messages to diverse audiences. Interactive workshops can help them practice delivering health education messages in culturally sensitive ways. Additionally, they should be trained to do communication channel assessments.

(e) *Psychosocial Support and Counselling*: As discussed earlier, many NTDs are associated with stigma, and millions of affected individuals live with mental health conditions and stigma associated with NTDs, which is often not paid enough attention by NTD programmes (Kuper, 2021). NTDs, like lymphatic filariasis and leishmaniasis, can cause physical disfigurements and disabilities, which, in addition to physical distress, can induce mental distress and stigma (World Health Organization, 2020a, b). While most programmes targeting NTD elimination focus on preventive strategies through MDA, the plight of the already affected is often ignored. The social work profession has a twofold significance in this regard. The community social work practice can engage in programmes that target the elimination of stigma associated with NTDs, and the clinical social work practice can engage in programmes that target the improvement of the mental health and psychological quality of life of the individuals affected by NTDs. This is a major gap in the current programmes for NTDs. While there are efforts to eliminate NTDs and research on the mental health implications of NTDs on the affected population, the interventions to mitigate adverse mental health effects are minimal, positioning social work as a key discipline in this regard. Therefore, social workers should be trained in providing psychosocial support, such as counselling, to address the emotional and mental health needs of the patients and their families. Training workshops on active listening, empathy and counselling techniques can help social workers develop these skills needed to provide effective psychosocial.

(f) *Advocacy Skills*: Health equity is a critical component when considering the case of NTDs. NTDs often involve a case of violation of human rights, particularly the right to health. Hence, rights-based interventions that address inequities in healthcare access, stigma and non-discrimination in health settings are considered relevant for the population affected by NTDs (Sun & Amon, 2018). Advocacy is a vital aspect of social work practice and aligns with the ethical principles of the profession, which can take the form of 'case advocacy' and 'cause advocacy' (Bull, 1989). The latter, i.e. cause advocacy, is employed to ensure social justice for larger sections of the society. Working with NTDs essentially involves working for the rights of communities that are marginalised and experience violations of the right to health. Social workers can act as social justice advocates who move beyond the immediate problem, i.e. the illness and advocate for changing social determinants that induce health inequity. The combination of advocacy and social action can effectively transform the social determinants of health for individuals affected by NTDs. Therefore, social workers should be equipped with advocacy skills to advocate for policy changes, resource allocation and social support systems to address the underlying social determinants of NTDs. Training can include sessions on advocacy strategies, policy analysis, engagement with policymakers, mobilising support and influencing decision-makers at various levels. Simulated advocacy campaigns and policy brief development exercises can help them practice advocacy skills for addressing NTD-related challenges.

(g) *Policy Practice*: In addition to advocacy, social workers must be trained in policy practice to engage in the policy-making process effectively. This involves understanding how policies are developed, implemented and evaluated and how social workers can influence policy to better address the needs of those affected by NTDs. Training should cover policy analysis, development of policy briefs and strategies for engaging with policymakers and stakeholders at various levels of government. India has implemented several policies and programs to address NTDs, with a focus on diseases such as lymphatic filariasis, dengue, leishmaniasis and leprosy. The National Vector Borne Disease Control Programme (NVBDCP) serves as a comprehensive initiative targeting vector-borne diseases. Additionally, there are disease-specific policies and programs in place, such as the National Leprosy Eradication Programme and the Accelerated Plan for Elimination of Lymphatic Filariasis, 2018. Social workers should be able to assess these existing policies' impact on NTD control and contribute to the creation of policies that promote equitable healthcare access. Workshops and simulations on policy practice can help social workers develop the skills necessary to influence policy and advocate for systemic changes.

(h) *Working as Interdisciplinary Team Members*: Working on NTDs is an interdisciplinary task, as NTDs are the outcome of a combination of biological, climatic and social factors. Hence, programmes for NTDs should essentially include professionals from multiple disciplines working together as a team. Social work professionals are trained to work in conjunction with other professionals, particularly medical professionals. This can improve the team's overall performance in terms of attaining the programme goals. Social workers, with their unique skills, can provide the team with unique insights into the situation, which might not immediately be visible to others. Social workers can help ensure that the programme and the team engage in culturally informed practices. Social workers, as interdisciplinary team members, can also provide insights to other team members, like clinicians, on the reluctance to seek treatment and how to address such problems. Social work professionals can engage as both clinical and community practitioners at the same time, adding depth to the team.

Social workers should be trained in interdisciplinary collaboration, communication and coordination to work effectively with diverse stakeholders and leverage their resources and expertise to address NTD-related challenges.

(i) *Research, Monitoring and Evaluation*: Social workers need expertise in research, monitoring, and evaluation to assess the effectiveness and impact of NTD control interventions and to make evidence-based decisions. Training should include skills in data collection methods, data analysis techniques and interpretation of findings. Practical training in quantitative and qualitative research methods, as well as using data analysis software, can help them build their capacity to work with NTD control missions.

(j) *Ethics*: As discussed earlier, adequate training is needed on ethical considerations when working with communities affected by NTDs. This includes understanding ethical dilemmas, navigating cultural differences and upholding professional standards of conduct.

The list of essential capacity-building domains, potential topics and methods are listed in Table 3.1. Each domain focuses on a specific area critical to the

Table 3.1 Capacity building of social workers engaged in NTD control programmes

No.	Capacity building domain	Topics	Methods
1	Epidemiology of NTDs	Disease transmission, causes, symptoms, treatment options, preventive measures and national programmes	Curriculum enhancement, interactive sessions, guest lectures and field visits
2	Cultural competence	Beliefs, practices, customs, healing practices and social structures of communities affected by NTD	Curriculum enhancement, lectures, simulation exercises and guest lectures
3	Community engagement and mobilisation	Interpersonal communication, relationship building, communication, and conducting meetings and discussions	Workshops, lectures, role-plays, case studies and field practicum
4	Health education and promotion	Health communication techniques and education materials	Lectures and hands-on workshops
5	Psychosocial support and counselling	Counselling techniques, listening and empathy	Lectures, workshops and field practicum
6	Advocacy skills	Advocacy strategies and policy analysis	Lectures, training and workshops
7	Policy practice	Policy analysis, development of policy briefs, and strategies for engaging with policymakers and stakeholders at various levels of government	Workshops, field practicum and simulations on policy practice
8	Inter-disciplinary collaboration	Networking, lobbying, communication and coordination	Lectures, workshops, role-plays and case-studies
9	Research, monitoring and evaluation	Data collection methods, data analysis techniques, report writing and information dissemination	Lectures, hands-on workshops, dissertation and mentoring
10	Ethics	Ethical considerations and professional standards	Lectures and role-play

effectiveness of social workers in NTD control, utilising a combination of theoretical and practical training methods to enhance their skills and knowledge.

3.6.1 Approaches for Capacity Building for Social Workers

Equipping social workers with the requisite skills and knowledge for effective NTD control necessitates a multifaceted approach that integrate both theoretical and practical aspects. Below are some strategies to achieve this:

(a) *Curriculum Enhancement*: Traditionally, the topic 'neglected tropical diseases' has been incorporated into life science or medical curricula such as MBBS, MD, zoology and entomology, while social work schools have largely overlooked these areas of the study even though these diseases carry significant impacts on communities. Therefore, educational institutions offering social work programmes can include modules on public health, including specific modules on diseases of poverty. These modules should cover topics such as the epidemiology of such diseases, social determinants of health, cultural competence, community engagement strategies, advocacy skills, ethical considerations and interdisciplinary collaboration. Moreover, institutions can add soft skills modules to their curriculum for training sessions on topics such as community engagement, health education, behaviour change communication, advocacy, data collection and trauma-informed care. These workshops can complement academic learning and provide students with practical skills for working in NTD control.

    Although many social work colleges in India offer medical social work as a specialisation, the majority of these programmes primarily focus on training students to deliver mental health services to individuals and families. Modules within these programmes often overlook NTDs and other diseases of poverty. Instead, the emphasis tends to be on topics such as assessment, diagnosis, therapies, and mental health legislation and policy. However, there are some exceptions, such as the Tata Institute of Social Sciences (TISS), which has recently introduced a course on social work in public health, which exclusively covers areas like health policies, programmes, legislations, health management and health research. Therefore, social work schools can create such programmes reflecting a broader perspective on addressing public health challenges beyond mental health concerns.

(b) *Field Practicum*: Field practicum is an integral component of social work curricula, allowing students to identify various issues affecting marginalised populations in society and implement innovative interventions at the grassroots level. Social work institutions can enhance these opportunities by incorporating field practicum or internships within national NTD national control programs such as the National Vector Borne Diseases Control Programme (NCVBDCP), National Centre for Disease Control (NCDC), or research institutes like the

Indian Council of Medical Research (ICMR), or NGO actively engaged in NTD control efforts. Additionally, students can gain hands-on experience by working alongside experienced health researchers or social work professionals who work for NTD-endemic areas and participating in community engagement activities, health education campaigns and advocacy initiatives. For this purpose, the institutions can enhance their collaborations with public health institutions, government agencies, non-governmental organisations (NGOs) and community-based organisations involved in NTD control. This can create opportunities for joint projects and fieldwork placements for students.

(c) *Workshops and Guest Lectures*: Social work schools can invite experts, practitioners, and researchers working in the field of NTD control to deliver guest lectures and conduct workshops for social work students. These sessions can provide valuable insights, practical examples and real-world perspectives on addressing NTDs in India. Additionally, such interactions can inspire students to consider field practicum, research projects and careers in public health.

(d) *Research*: Faculties in social work schools can encourage their students to undertake research projects related to NTDs. This can help students develop critical thinking skills, research methodology proficiency and a deeper understanding of the social determinants of health and disease. Importantly, faculty members should also be trained in designing and implementing research studies in public health.

(e) *Field Visits*: Observation visits are an integral component of social work education in India, offering students opportunities to visit and engage directly with communities and social service organisations. Students often visit government institutions, NGOs and communities in their first or second semesters to become familiar with their academic areas. The social work schools can organise field visits to NTD-endemic areas, health facilities and community-based organisations involved in NTD control initiatives. These experiences can help students gain first-hand knowledge of NTD control and understand the challenges faced by the health system.

3.7 Social Work Research for the Cause of NTDs

It is widely acknowledged that social work practice should be guided by scientific research (Erbay, 2017). When employing interventions to solve large-scale problems, the profession must advance the evidence base regarding which interventions are effective in what settings, when and with whom (Proctor, 2017). Furthermore, there is a need for the profession to progress by developing and testing new tools and innovative interventions through a concreted research process. Additionally, the concept of the scientific practitioner within the social work profession has recently gained much appreciation. They are practitioners who integrate practice with research, considering research as a tool to be used in practice (Bloom, 1975; Fischer, 1978). These practitioners often utilise research evidence to select interventions, collect data from the field and do empirical analysis to see whether the interventions are effective for specific populations in given contexts (Blythe, 1992). Therefore, the role of a scientific practitioner is particularly important in addressing NTDs due to the complex socio-economic and cultural factors contributing to the spread of the disease.

Social science researchers involved in NTD research often focus on studies examining various social factors perpetuating the cycle of NTD transmission (Shrivastava & Shrivastava, 2013). They support programme-implementing agencies in developing targeted interventions addressing the social causes of NTDs, thereby enhancing the effectiveness of control programs. In addition, their research facilitates community engagement and empowerment, ensuring culturally appropriate and sustainable interventions (Molyneux et al., 2018). Importantly, the findings from social science research have a huge impact on policy decisions for NTDs control at local, national and international levels.

However, conducting social work research in the context of NTDs poses many challenges. It is interdisciplinary, requiring collaboration with healthcare professionals, epidemiologists, and entomologists due to the complex interplay between social, environmental and biological factors involved in NTD transmission. Additionally, social workers conducting research in this area need adequate knowledge about disease transmission and training in health research concepts and methodologies.

Social work research in the context of NTDs in India can cover a wide range of topics and areas. A list of topics for NTD social work research is listed in Fig. 3.3 and explained below.

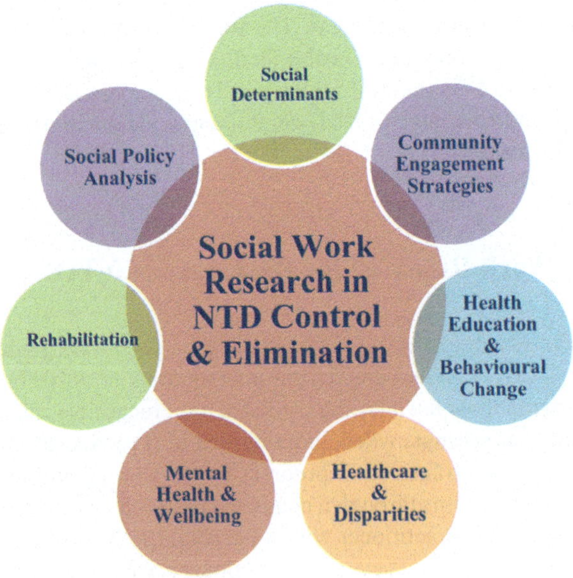
Social Determinants
Community Engagement Strategies
Health Education & Behavioural Change
Healthcare & Disparities
Mental Health & Wellbeing
Rehabilitation
Social Policy Analysis
Social Work Research in NTD Control & Elimination

Fig. 3.3 Areas of social work research in NTDs control

(a) *Social Determinants*: Social workers may focus on research to understand the social determinants which largely contribute to the spread and persistence of NTDs in India. Additionally, behavioural risk factors in endemic areas are frequently documented. Given India's vast cultural diversity, evidence from such research can aid in designing tailored behavioural interventions addressing the specific needs of communities residing in different areas. Current social science research endeavours are mainly focused on identifying how social determinants such as poverty, inadequate housing, lack of education and healthcare accessibility, intersectionality, community behaviour and social structure shape NTD transmission in the country. For instance, several studies have covered socio-economic status, behavioural aspects, housing structures, sanitation and cultural aspects of NTDs (Delmelle et al., 2016; Farinelli et al., 2018; Upadhyayula et al., 2012; Vijay Kumar & Ramaiah, 2008).

(b) *Community Engagement Strategies*: Another important area of research for social workers in NTD control is exploring strategies for engaging communities in disease control efforts. This involves designing and implementing novel strategies to promote community participation in disease control and prevention. Additionally, social workers can engage in research to empower local populations to take ownership of preventive measures and build the capacity of local healthcare workers and community leaders in NTD control. For instance, much research has examined the association between community participation and empowerment strategies and NTD outcomes (Krentel et al., 2021; Njomo et al., 2020; Silumbwe et al., 2019; Sulistyawati et al., 2019).

(c) *Health Education and Behaviour Change*: Social workers are also involved in research to implement and evaluate the effectiveness of certain health education interventions for the control of NTDs in disease-endemic communities. They may do intervention studies to test new health educational tools or evaluate the existing system for behaviour change communication to support the promotion of preventive behaviour among communities. For instance, studies have been conducted to assess the impact of educational interventions on NTD control (Kusuma et al., 2019; Nandha & Krishnamoorthy, 2012; Roja et al., 2022).

(d) *Healthcare and Disparities*: Another potential area for social work researchers in this area is the examination of facilitators and barriers to accessing healthcare services among communities affected by NTDs. This can include the evaluation of barriers to healthcare services, gaps in service delivery and supply chain, and the cost of illness. Notably, previous studies have reported the significant impact of healthcare accessibility on an individual's health-seeking behaviour (Guntur et al., 2022; Orish et al., 2021). Therefore, research in this area helps improve healthcare delivery and accessibility, especially in underserved areas. Many studies in India have explored these aspects (Chawla, 2023; Kusuma et al., 2019; Sawers & Stillwaggon, 2020).

(e) *Mental Health and Well-Being*: Research in this area could explore the mental health challenges faced by individuals affected by NTDs in India and assess the psychosocial impact of these diseases on patients, their families and communities. Previous research has found a significant impact of certain NTDs on patients and their families. For instance, it has been reported that the physical morbidity resulting from lymphedema and hydrocele due to LF, coupled with the social stigma, creates considerable psychological distress among patients. Therefore, social workers could carry out studies on the prevalence of depression, anxiety, stigma and discrimination among patients, as well as identify coping mechanisms and resilience factors. Additionally, research could evaluate the effectiveness of mental health interventions and support services for enhancing the well-being and quality of life of NTD patients.

(f) *Rehabilitation*: Research in this area could focus on the rehabilitation needs of individuals affected by NTDs, particularly in terms of physical, social and vocational rehabilitation. As discussed earlier, some NTDs lead to physical challenges. For instance, leprosy remains a leading cause of peripheral neuropathy and disability in the world. Studies could examine the barriers to accessing rehabilitation services and assess the effectiveness of existing rehabilitation programs in India. Additionally, research could explore innovative approaches to rehabilitation, including community-based rehabilitation initiatives and peer support networks. Evaluative research could measure the impact of rehabilitation interventions on the overall well-being of NTD patients.

(g) *Social Policy Analysis*: Social workers could focus on research that critically analyses the social policies and programs related to NTD control and prevention in India. Studies could examine the policy landscape governing NTDs, including government strategies, funding allocations, and intersectoral collaboration mechanisms. In India, numerous disease-specific programmes and policies like the accelerated strategy for LF elimination 2018, the national leprosy eradication programme and deworming programmes against STH are operational. Social workers can carry out specific operational and implementation research to solve various challenges and gaps in the existing policy execution and identify opportunities for policy reform and advocacy. Comparative policy analyses could be conducted to draw lessons from other countries' approaches to NTD control and prevention, informing evidence-based policy recommendations for India.

3.7.1 Research Methods for Social Workers in NTD Control

Social work research on neglected tropical diseases (NTDs) in India has access to a range of methodological approaches to gain insights into the factors associated with these diseases. While quantitative cross-sectional surveys offer extensive coverage of various aspects of diseases, qualitative methodologies, such as in-depth interviews and focus group discussions, provide valuable avenues for capturing the lived experiences and perceptions of individuals affected by NTDs. Moreover, mixed-methods research designs present an opportunity to gather both quantitative data on disease outcomes and qualitative insights into patients' experiences and perspectives, providing a more holistic understanding of the impact of NTDs and the effectiveness of intervention strategies.

Qualitative research is essential for understanding NTDs within the specific context of India due to its ability to provide in-depth insights into the intersectionality of various social, cultural, economic and environmental factors influencing disease outcomes. Several recent qualitative studies, both in India and globally, have delved into various aspects of NTDs (Adhikari et al., 2015; Kumar et al., 2023; Taylor et al., 2022). For instance, a recent qualitative study in Ethiopia utilised semi-structured interviews and focus group discussions to examine the impact of leprosy, podoconiosis and lymphatic filariasis on family quality of life, revealing significant challenges like participation restrictions, reduced productivity, stigma and mental health issues affecting both patients and their families (Van't Noordende et al., 2020). Similarly, qualitative studies conducted in Odisha, India, through focus group discussions, aimed to understand the experiences of individuals with lymphedema. These studies highlighted the social, physical and economic hurdles faced by patients, including issues related to marriage and social stigma associated with NTDs (Cassidy et al., 2016).

Moreover, participatory research holds significant potential in India for studying NTDs, offering opportunities to effectively engage with various stakeholders such as policymakers, healthcare providers, programme officials and community members in planning and executing NTD programmes. A notable example of such research is the school-based NTD intervention studies. For instance, research conducted in Chennai involved school children in dengue control through participatory group activities and demonstrations, highlighting the efficacy of participatory approaches in NTD prevention (Roja et al., 2022). Another example is the community-based dengue control intervention study in Delhi in 2011, where quasi-experimental research was conducted using participatory approaches such as accelerated community mobilisation by organising meetings of representatives of resident welfare associations (RWAs), trade unions, school teachers and children, municipal councillors and local opinion leaders for dengue control (Nagpal et al., 2016). Furthermore, social workers can carry out specific operational and implementation research to solve various challenges and gaps in the existing policy execution and identify opportunities for policy reform and advocacy. Overall, by employing a combination of qualitative, participatory, mixed-methods and implementation research approaches, social workers can significantly contribute to advancing knowledge and informing evidence-based practices for NTD control and prevention in India.

3.8 Case Studies of NTD Programmes and the Role of Social Work

Several NTD programmes have been implemented in India and globally, aiming to alleviate the burden of these diseases on affected populations. Within India, various national-level agencies, independent research organisations and individual researchers have implemented numerous initiatives to control NTDs. The following section discusses two case studies focusing on leprosy and lymphatic filariasis, which exemplify the role of social workers in combating these diseases.

Cannon (1964) demonstrated the application of a social casework approach in supporting individuals affected by Hansen's disease, commonly known as leprosy. Drawing upon his extensive experiences and observations in social work within public health settings, he emphasised the broader implication of social casework in the holistic care of Hansen's disease patients. His approach involved assessments of patients' social and familial backgrounds, facilitating communication and rapport-building between patients and their families, providing counselling and emotional support and assisting with vocational rehabilitation and reintegration into society. He highlighted the significant impact of social casework on the well-being and quality of life of the patients. Addressing the social and psychological dimensions of their illness contributed to the overall effectiveness of medical treatment and rehabilitation efforts of the patients. Additionally, his method significantly contributed to minimising the stigma and social isolation experienced by leprosy patients in his intervention, thereby promoting their social integration and acceptance within their communities.

Nandha and Krishnamoorthy (2012) implemented a community-based intervention to accelerate the elimination of lymphatic filariasis (LF) in Tamil Nadu, India. The team employed a mixed-methods approach, combining socio-behavioural educational interventions, community-based vector control measures and impact assessment. The team devised and implemented community-based education campaigns to raise awareness about lymphatic filariasis, its transmission, prevention methods and the importance of community involvement in vector control. They actively organised and mobilised local community members for vector control interventions such as mosquito bed net distribution, larval source management and indoor residual spraying, as well as providing education and support. Finally, they assessed the impact of these interventions on the prevalence and transmission of LF and collected extensive quantitative and qualitative data, such as community perceptions and behaviours related to LF prevention, as well as the social and cultural factors influencing health outcomes.

These case studies highlight the significant roles that social workers play in combating NTDs such as LF and leprosy. These diseases continue to pose significant public health challenges in India. Social workers can employ a spectrum of approaches, as evidenced in these case studies, from individual-based casework to large-scale community-based interventions to support both patients and government efforts in NTD control. Moreover, these case studies emphasise the need for multidisciplinary approaches, where social workers collaborate with healthcare professionals, entomologists and communities.

3.9 Conclusion

This chapter sheds light on the imperative role of social work in addressing neglected tropical diseases (NTDs). Despite the historical lack of emphasis on social work within NTD interventions, it is evident that the profession's principles and practices align closely with NTD prevention and management. Proposing a new social work model for NTD control, the chapter advocates for a more holistic approach to NTD interventions that acknowledges the socio-economic and cultural dimensions of these diseases. By equipping social work graduates with the necessary knowledge, skills and competencies, they can play a crucial role in addressing the complex challenges associated with NTDs in India and contribute to improving the health and well-being of affected communities. Additionally, social work research in the context of NTDs is vital for understanding the social determinants of disease transmission, designing effective interventions, promoting community engagement and addressing healthcare disparities. Through research, social workers can contribute valuable evidence to inform policy decisions and improve NTD control efforts in India.

References

Adams, R. (2017). *Empowerment, participation and social work*. Bloomsbury Publishing.

Adams, A. M., Vuckovic, M., Birch, E., Brant, T. A., Bialek, S., Yoon, D., Koroma, J., Direny, A., Shott, J., Lemoine, J. F., Dembele, M., & Baker, M. C. (2018). Eliminating neglected tropical diseases in urban areas: A review of challenges, strategies and research directions for successful mass drug administration. *Tropical medicine and infectious disease, 3*(4), 122. https://doi.org/10.3390/tropicalmed3040122

Addiss, D. G., Kienast, Y., & Lavery, J. V. (2021). Ethical dimensions of neglected tropical disease programming. *Transactions of the Royal Society of Tropical Medicine and Hygiene, 115*(2), 190–195.

Adhikari, R. K., Sherchand, J. B., Mishra, S. R., Ranabhat, K., Pokharel, A., Devkota, P., Mishra, D., Ghimire, Y. C., Gelal, K., Paudel, R., & Wagle, R. R. (2015). Health-seeking behaviors and self-care practices of people with filarial lymphoedema in Nepal: A qualitative study. *Journal of Tropical Medicine, 2015*, 260359. https://doi.org/10.1155/2015/260359

Allotey, P., Reidpath, D. D., & Pokhrel, S. (2010). Social sciences research in neglected tropical diseases 1: The ongoing neglect in the neglected tropical diseases. *Health research policy and systems, 8*(32), 1–8.

Attree, P., French, B., Milton, B., Povall, S., Whitehead, M., & Popay, J. (2011). The experience of community engagement for individuals: A rapid review of evidence. *Health & Social Care in the Community, 19*(3), 250–260.

Babu, B. V., & Babu, G. R. (2014). Coverage of, and compliance with, mass drug administration under the programme to eliminate lymphatic filariasis in India: A systematic review. *Transactions of the Royal Society of Tropical Medicine and Hygiene, 108*(9), 538–549.

Baikady, R., Cheng, S. L., & Channaveer, R. M. (2021). Eight decades of existence and search for an identity: Educators perspectives on social work education in contemporary India. *Social Work Education, 40*(8), 994–1009.

Bailey, F., Eaton, J., Jidda, M., van Brakel, W. H., Addiss, D. G., & Molyneux, D. H. (2019). Neglected tropical diseases and mental health: progress, partnerships, and integration. *Trends in Parasitology, 35*(1), 23–31.

Baldock, P. (1974). *Community work and social work* (pp. 66–82). Routledge & Kegan Paul.

Banerjee, S., & Varma, R. P. (2013). Factors affecting non-adherence among patients diagnosed with unipolar depression in a psychiatric Department of a Tertiary Hospital in Kolkata, India. *Depression Research and Treatment, 2013*, 809542. https://doi.org/10.1155/2013/809542

Banerjee, S., Bandyopadhyay, K., Khan, M. F., Akkilagunta, S., Selvaraj, K., Tripathy, J. P., et al. (2019). Coverage of mass drug administration for elimination of lymphatic filariasis in urban Nagpur, Central India: A mixed method study. *Journal of Family Medicine and Primary Care, 8*(9), 3009–3014.

Bloom, M. (1975). *The paradox of helping: Introduction to the philosophy of scientific practice*. Wiley.

Blue, S., Shove, E., Carmona, C., & Kelly, M. P. (2016). Theories of practice and public health: understanding (un)healthy practices. *Critical Public Health, 26*(1), 36–50.

Blythe, B. (1992). Should undergraduate and graduate social work students be taught to conduct empirically based practice? Yes! *Journal of Social Work Education, 2*(3), 260–263.

Bull, D. (1989). The social worker's advocacy role: A British quest for a Canadian perspective. *Canadian Social Work Review/Revue canadienne de service social, 6*(1), 49–68.

Cannon, W. E. (1964). Social casework for patients with Hansen's disease. *Public Health Reports, 79*(3), 193–199.

Cassidy, T., Worrell, C. M., Little, K., Prakash, A., Patra, I., Rout, J., & Fox, L. M. (2016). Experiences of a community-based Lymphedema management program for lymphatic Filariasis in Odisha state, India: An analysis of focus group discussions with patients, families, community members and program volunteers. *PLoS Neglected Tropical Diseases, 10*(2), e0004424. https://doi.org/10.1371/journal.pntd.0004424

CDC. (2023). *Neglected tropical diseases*. Available at: https://www.cdc.gov/globalhealth/ntd/resources/ntd_factsheet_2023.pdf

Chandra, A., Sreeganga, S. D., Rath, N., & Ramaprasad, A. (2023). Healthcare policies to eliminate neglected tropical diseases (NTDs) in India: A roadmap. *International Journal of Environmental Research and Public Health, 20*(19), 6842. https://doi.org/10.3390/ijerph20196842

Chawla, N. S. (2023). Unveiling the ABCs: Identifying India's healthcare service gaps. *Cureus, 15*(7), e42398. https://doi.org/10.7759/cureus.42398

Chitereka, C. (2009). Social work in a developing continent: The case of Africa. *Advances in Social Work, 10*(2), 144–156.

Coulton, C. (2005). The place of community in social work practice research: Conceptual and methodological developments. *Social Work Research, 29*(2), 73–86.

Delmelle, E., Hagenlocher, M., Kienberger, S., & Casas, I. (2016). A spatial model of socioeconomic and environmental determinants of dengue fever in Cali, Colombia. *Acta Tropica, 164*, 169–176. https://doi.org/10.1016/j.actatropica.2016.08.028

Erbay, Ercüment (2017). Importance of research in social work practice: A pilot study from Turkey. *Journal of Social Service Research, 43*(3), 395–403.

Farinelli, E. C., Baquero, O. S., Stephan, C., & Chiaravalloti-Neto, F. (2018). Low socioeconomic condition and the risk of dengue fever: A direct relationship. *Acta Tropica, 180*, 47–57. https://doi.org/10.1016/j.actatropica.2018.01.005

Fischer, J. (1978). *Effective casework practice: An eclectic approach*. McGraw-Hill.

Gangrade, K. D. (1971). *Community organisation in India*. Popular Prakashan.

Garapati, P., Pal, B., Siddiqui, N. A., Bimal, S., Das, P., Murti, K., & Pandey, K. (2018). Knowledge, stigma, health seeking behaviour and its determinants among patients with post kalaazar dermal leishmaniasis, Bihar, India. *PLoS One, 13*(9), e0203407. https://doi.org/10.1371/journal.pone.0203407

Guntur, R. D., Kingsley, J., & Islam, F. M. A. (2022). Malaria treatment-seeking behaviour and its associated factors: A cross-sectional study in rural East Nusa Tenggara Province, Indonesia. *PLoS One, 17*(2), e0263178. https://doi.org/10.1371/journal.pone.0263178

Harper, E. B., & Dunham, A. (1959). *Community organisation in action*. Association Press.

ICMR. (2003, October). *Health status of primitive tribes of Orissa* (Vol. 33, No. 10). Available at: https://main.icmr.nic.in/sites/default/files/icmr_bulletins/BUOCT03.pdf

IFSW. (2018). *Global social work statement of ethical principles*. Available at: https://www.ifsw.org/global-social-work-statement-of-ethical-principles/?hub=main

Indian Council of Medical Research (ICMR). (2017). *National ethical guidelines for biomedical and health research involving human participants*. Available at: https://ethics.ncdirindia.org/asset/pdf/ICMR_National_Ethical_Guidelines.pdf. Accessed 27 Jan 2024.

Krentel, A., Gyapong, M., McFarland, D. A., Ogundahunsi, O., Titaley, C. R., & Addiss, D. G. (2021). Keeping communities at the Centre of efforts to eliminate lymphatic filariasis: Learning from the past to reach a future free of lymphatic filariasis. *International Health, 13*(1), 55–59.

Kumar, P., Ahmad, S., Bhar, D., Roy, R., & Singh, B. (2023). "Whenever I tell her to wear slippers, she turns a deaf ear. She never listens": A qualitative descriptive research on the barriers to basic lymphedema management and quality of life in lymphatic filariasis patients in a rural block of eastern India. *Parasites & Vectors, 16*(1), 429. https://doi.org/10.1186/s13071-023-06036-0

Kumari, A. K., Harichandrakumar, K. T., Krishnamoorthy, K., & Das, L. K. (2010). The stigmata and discrimination experienced, in southern India, by cases of lymphatic filariasis. *Annals of Tropical Medicine & Parasitology, 104*(5), 421–426.

Kuper, H. (2021). Disability, mental health, stigma and discrimination and neglected tropical diseases. *Transactions of the Royal Society of Tropical Medicine and Hygiene, 115*(2), 145–146.

Kusuma, Y. S., Burman, D., Kumari, R., Lamkang, A. S., & Babu, B. V. (2019). Impact of health education based intervention on community's awareness of dengue and its prevention in Delhi, India. *Global Health Promotion, 26*(1), 50–59.

Molyneux, D. H., Dean, L., Adekeye, O., Stothard, J. R., & Theobald, S. (2018). The changing global landscape of health and disease: Addressing challenges and opportunities for sustaining progress towards control and elimination of neglected tropical diseases (NTDs). *Parasitology, 145*(13), 1647–1654.

Nagpal, B. N., Gupta, S. K., Shamim, A., Vikram, K., Srivastava, A., Tuli, N. R., Saxena, R., Singh, H., Singh, V. P., Bhagat, V. N., Yadav, N. K., & Valecha, N. (2016). Control of Aedes aegypti breeding: A novel intervention for prevention and control of dengue in an endemic zone of Delhi, India. *PLoS One, 11*(12), e0166768. https://doi.org/10.1371/journal.pone.0166768

Nandha, B., & Krishnamoorthy, K. (2012). Impact of education campaign on community-based vector control in hastening the process of elimination of lymphatic filariasis in Tamil Nadu, South India. *Health Education Research, 27*(4), 585–594.

NAPSW. (2015). *Code of ethics for professional social workers in India*. Available at: https://www.napswi.org/pdf/NAPSWI_Code_of_Ethics).pdf

National Association of Social Workers. (2024). *Code of ethics*. Available at: https://www.socialworkers.org/About/Ethics/Code-of-Ethics/Code-of-Ethics-English

Njomo, D. W., Kibe, L. W., Kimani, B. W., Okoyo, C., Omondi, W. P., & Sultani, H. M. (2020). Addressing barriers of community participation and access to mass drug administration for lymphatic filariasis elimination in Coastal Kenya using a participatory approach. *PLoS Neglected Tropical Diseases, 14*(9), e0008499. https://doi.org/10.1371/journal.pntd.0008499

Orish, V. N., Maalman, R. S. E., Donkor, O. Y., Ceruantes, B. Y. H., Osei, E., Amu, H., et al. (2021). Assessing health-seeking behaviour and malaria prevention practices among communities in four districts of the Volta Region of Ghana. *Malaria Journal, 20*, 1–13. https://doi.org/10.1186/s12936-021-03986-7

Popay, J., Attree, P., Hornby, D., Milton, B., Whitehead, M., French, B., et al. (2007). *Community engagement in initiatives addressing the wider social determinants of health: A rapid review of evidence on impact, experience and process*. University of Lancaster. Available at: https://www.nice.org.uk/guidance/ph9/documents/social-determinants-evidence-review-final2. Accessed 1 July 2020.

Proctor, E. (2017). The pursuit of quality for social work practice: Three generations and counting. *Journal of the Society for Social Work and Research, 8*(3), 335–353.

Reamer, F. (2006). *Social work values and ethics* (3rd ed.). Colombia University Press.

Roja, C., Lakshmi, A. S., Rani, M. A., Eapen, A., Chokkara, R., & Avudaiappan, S. L. (2022). Effect of school-based educational interventions on the knowledge of malaria and dengue among higher secondary school children in Chennai, India: A pre and post-intervention study. *Cureus, 14*(7). https://doi.org/10.7759/cureus.26536

Ross, M. G. (1967). *Community organisation*. Harper and Row.

Ruth, B. J., & Marshall, J. W. (2017). A history of social work in public health. *American Journal of Public Health, 107*(3), 236–242.

Saha, S., Chauhan, A., Hamlai, M., Saiyad, V., Makwana, S., Shah, K., & Pandya, A. (2021). Unique collaboration of modern medicine and traditional faith-healing for the treatment of mental illness: Best practice from Gujarat. *Journal of Family Medicine and Primary Care, 10*(1), 521–526.

Sawers, L., & Stillwaggon, E. (2020). Economic costs and benefits of community-based lymphedema-management programs for lymphatic filariasis in India. *The American Journal of Tropical Medicine and Hygiene, 103*(1), 295–302.

Shrivastava, S. R., & Shrivastava, P. S. (2013). Targeting neglected tropical diseases in India: Some recent developments. *Journal of Research in Medical Sciences: Journal of Isfahan University of Medical Sciences, 18*(1), 73–74.

Silumbwe, A., Halwindi, H., & Zulu, J. M. (2019). How community engagement strategies shape participation in mass drug administration programmes for lymphatic filariasis: The case of Luangwa District, Zambia. *PLoS Neglected Tropical Diseases, 13*(11), e0007861. https://doi.org/10.1371/journal.pntd.0007861

Sulistyawati, S., Dwi Astuti, F., Rahmah Umniyati, S., Tunggul Satoto, T. B., Lazuardi, L., Nilsson, M., et al. (2019). Dengue vector control through community empowerment: Lessons learned from a community-based study in Yogyakarta, Indonesia. *International Journal of Environmental Research and Public Health, 16*(6), 1013. https://doi.org/10.3390/ijerph16061013

Sun, N., & Amon, J. J. (2018). Addressing inequity: Neglected tropical diseases and human rights. *Health and Human Rights, 20*(1), 11–25.

Taylor, M., Thomas, R., Oliver, S., & Garner, P. (2022). Community views on mass drug administration for filariasis: A qualitative evidence synthesis. *The Cochrane Database of Systematic Reviews, 2*(2), CD013638. https://doi.org/10.1002/14651858.CD013638.pub2

Upadhyayula, S. M., Mutheneni, S. R., Kadiri, M. R., Kumaraswamy, S., & Nagalla, B. (2012). A cohort study of lymphatic filariasis on socio economic conditions in Andhra Pradesh, India. *PLoS One, 7*(3), e33779. https://doi.org/10.1371/journal.pone.0033779

van't Noordende, A. T., Aycheh, M. W., & Schippers, A. (2020). The impact of leprosy, podoconiosis and lymphatic filariasis on family quality of life: A qualitative study in Northwest Ethiopia. *PLoS Neglected Tropical Diseases, 14*(3), e0008173. https://doi.org/10.1371/journal.pntd.0008173

Vijay Kumar, K. N., & Ramaiah, K. D. (2008). Usage of personal-protection measures against mosquitoes and the low prevalences of Wuchereria bancrofti microfilaraemia in the Indian city of Chennai. *Annals of Tropical Medicine & Parasitology, 102*(5), 391–397.

World Health Organization. (2007). *Promoting safety of medicines for children*. World Health Organization.

World Health Organization. (2010). *Working to overcome the global impact of neglected tropical diseases: First WHO report on neglected tropical diseases* (Vol. 1). Available from: http://whqlibdoc.who.int/publications/2010/9789241564090_eng.pdf

World Health Organization. (2019). *Preventive chemotherapy: tools for improving the quality of reported data and information: A field manual for implementation*. Available at: https://www.who.int/publications/i/item/9789241516464

World Health Organization. (2020a). *Community engagement: A health promotion guide for universal health coverage in the hands of the people*. Available at: https://www.who.int/publications/i/item/9789240010529

World Health Organization. (2020b). *Mental health of people with neglected tropical diseases: towards a person-centred approach*. Retrieved from https://iris.who.int/bitstream/handle/10665/335885/9789240004528-eng.pdf

World Health Organization. (2021). *Neglected tropical diseases*. Retrieved from https://www.who.int/health-topics/neglected-tropical-diseases

Chapter 4
Towards Sustainable Impact: Future Directions in Social Work for NTD Control and Elimination

4.1 Introduction

As discussed in the previous chapters, neglected tropical diseases (NTDs) pose a formidable barrier to the achievement of global health equity, affecting the most vulnerable among the global population. These diseases, often endemic in low-resource settings, perpetuate cycles of poverty, suffering and disability, hindering progress towards health and development goals. The global agenda for the control and elimination of NTDs revolves around preventive medical approaches like mass drug administration. While medical interventions dominate the discourse, they often overlook the pivotal role of social determinants on the distribution and impact of NTDs within communities. Despite its strengths in addressing the social determinants of NTDs, the social work profession is often relegated as a 'non-essential discipline' in many NTD programmes, undermining its potential to address the structural factors driving NTD transmission and persistence. Consequently, social workers find themselves on the periphery, struggling to assert their expertise and contribute meaningfully to NTD control efforts. As it stands now, social work occupies a precarious position in terms of NTD control and elimination efforts. While the efficacy of social work discipline in addressing the social determinants of health is widely acknowledged, the recognition and integration of the social work profession into NTD initiatives still remain limited.

While it is to be acknowledged that medical interventions like MDA have been effective in the control and elimination of NTDs to a great extent, a segment of the endemic population does not adhere to such preventive efforts due to health system distrust, poor knowledge and other socio-cultural elements (Taylor et al., 2022; Mitchell et al., 2022). Given the dwindling compliance to MDA and the evolving community dynamics, ensuring people's participation is a task that requires specialised efforts. Social work can address this critical gap in preventive public health interventions effectively. Social workers possess skills and expertise in building

© The Author(s), under exclusive license to Springer Nature Switzerland AG 2024

M. Jabir, A. C. Choolayil, *Social Work with Populations Vulnerable to Neglected Tropical Diseases*, SpringerBriefs in Social Work,
https://doi.org/10.1007/978-3-031-68997-0_4

trust, fostering dialogue and empowering communities to take ownership of health programmes. By leveraging these strengths, social workers can play a pivotal role in overcoming barriers to participation and promoting sustainable behaviour change within endemic communities. However, despite its strengths in facilitating NTD control and prevention through efforts to engage communities, the role of social work is often unrecognised. This chapter, drawing from the previous chapter, briefly summarises the challenges faced by social work professionals in the domain of NTD control and prevention programmes and lays out future directions for the profession.

4.2 The Challenges in Positioning NTD Social Work as an Essential Profession

As discussed, the profession of social work is often not acknowledged as an essential profession in NTD control and elimination programmes. This is not surprising given that professional social work in general, despite long-term efforts, has failed to establish itself as a recognised profession in India. The challenges related to establishing social work as a recognised profession in India start right from the domain of social work education. Despite the introduction of professional social work education in India as early as 1936, the system of education is still reliant on Western approaches despite longstanding calls for indigenisation. The social work ecosystem in India lacks a proper definition, lacks a regulatory framework, has a vast diversity among the schools and lacks the lack professional identity (Baikady et al., 2020). The idea of regulating social work and establishing a National Council for Social Work Education was proposed as early as 1980 by the University Grants Commission (UGC), which is the apex statutory authority responsible for regulating the standards of higher education in India (Mathew, 2020). However, the National Council is still not established despite the National Council of Social Work (education and practice) Bill getting circulated in 2020. This lack of recognition of social work as a professional discipline and the absence of a regulatory body have impacted social work education and practice in India adversely, denying it the recognition and importance it deserves. This has, in turn, affected how social work practice in specific settings is recognised by the state mechanism as well as the community, including in the case of NTD social work. This section lists a set of challenges that the social work profession faces due to external dynamics and from within the profession in establishing itself as a relevant profession, specifically in the context of NTDs.

(a) *Under-recognised Role in Public Health*: Despite the fact that the social work profession has emphasised its role in the public health domain from the very early stages (Ruth & Marshall, 2017), the role in NTD control and prevention is rather unrecognised. This limited recognition of the social work profession, despite the wide acknowledgement of its importance, can be attributed to several factors. The primary limitation that restricts the role of social work in NTD interventions, as discussed earlier, is the absence of clear delineation and recognition within public health frameworks due to a disproportionate emphasis on medical interventions. Also, social sciences disciplines are often labelled homogenously under a single umbrella in most public health research with poor recognition of the unique skill and knowledge base of individual disciplines (Allotey et al., 2010). Social work, a practice-based discipline, is often equated with academic disciplines, thereby understating its importance. This understatement of the relevance of the social work discipline in the context of the public health domain, particularly NTD programmes, means that social work interventions are considered non-essential.

(b) *Limited Research and Evidence*: NTD social work is not well documented in the literature, given the fact that NTDs themselves started gaining attention only in the past couple of decades (Molyneux et al., 2021). Also given the fact that the social work literature itself was mostly Western until recently (Fleming et al., 2023) and NTDs were prevalent in developing countries in Asia and Africa, there are limited documentation of NTD social work. Despite social workers engaging in NTD control and prevention activities in low- and middle-income countries, there is limited documentation on the nature and role of NTD social work. This could be due to a lack of academic interest in NTD social work and/or a limited number of practitioners engaging in NTD social work. The end product is very few records and guidelines on the role and nature of NTD social work. Also, there is limited research and evidence for the effectiveness of social work interventions for NTDs in comparison with medical interventions. While medical interventions like MDA can provide data that showcases visible changes, social work interventions are often qualitative, involving methods to ensure community participation to accelerate control and elimination, often complementing the medical interventions. These changes are often qualitative and cannot be quantified but contribute immensely to the success of NTD programmes. The lesser visible quantitative outcomes paired with the poor social work infrastructure in most developing countries can hinder the efforts to project social work as an essential discipline in NTD control and prevention. Social workers may struggle to demonstrate the impact of their interventions and make a compelling case for their inclusion in NTD control efforts.

(c) *Lack of Social Work Infrastructure*: Another limitation in projecting NTD social work as a professional practice is the poor recognition of the social work profession as a whole and the lack of professional organisations in most developing countries. For instance, social work education and practice face the challenge of a lack of recognition in most Asian (Nikku & Pulla, 2014) and African countries (Chitereka, 2009). There are continued efforts to establish regional regulatory bodies across the globe but it is still a work in progress (Ioakimidis & Sookraj, 2021). This is one of the most important structural barriers in the global context when it comes to the recognition of social work as an essential discipline in NTD programmes. Most NTDs are endemic in low- and middle-income countries where social work infrastructure is, in most cases, a work in progress.

Many nations do not have state-recognised professional organisations that can argue for the case of professional social work. This lack of social work infrastructure and limited recognition from the state mechanisms are limitations in advocating for NTD social work in most developing countries that are endemic to NTDs. In addition, limited resources in middle- and low-income countries can result in the prioritisation of standalone medical interventions without giving adequate importance to community dynamics. However, such approaches can impact the success of MDA programmes since social determinants influence adherence to MDA drives (Mitchell et al., 2022).

(d) *Demarcation of Community and Medical Social Work*: The disproportionate emphasis on medical interventions is not the only reason for the limited recognition of the social work profession. The existing landscape of social work practice presents its own set of challenges. The first and foremost involves the demarcation of community and medical social work practices. The division between medical social work and community social work creates silos, hindering collaboration and coordination. While specialisations are beneficial, generalist practices provide a holistic picture to address the situation comprehensively (Blom, 2004). The perception that medical social workers are committed to clinical settings involving individual-level care and community social workers are committed to broader community-level interventions restricts the holistic scope of social work practice. Bridging this divide and practising an integrated approach leveraging the strengths of community social work and medical social work could be a starting point in projecting social work as an essential profession in controlling and preventing NTDs.

(e) *Funding Limitations*: Since most countries endemic to NTDs are in the low- to middle-income spectrum, there is limited financial allocation for healthcare in general, and in extension, NTD control and prevention programmes are allocated with limited resources. This limited availability of resources often makes the health system rely solely on pharmacological interventions, with limited emphasis on social determinants. This is a major constraint in pairing social work interventions with pharmacological interventions in most developing countries, thereby limiting the role of NTD social work.

Addressing these challenges requires a concerted effort from the social work community. By investing in social work infrastructure, promoting interdisciplinary collaboration, raising awareness of the profession's role and contributions and addressing systemic inequalities, the effectiveness of NTD control efforts can be enhanced. This key message should be disseminated to key stakeholders and should be advocated. The next section deals with the steps to be taken to advocate and promote NTD social work.

4.3 Future Directions in Establishing NTD Social Work as an Essential Practice

One of the fundamental arguments in the discourse of NTD control and prevention is the need to attain health equity. NTDs disproportionately affect people with limited resources and exacerbate health inequity. Addressing these inequities in health involves addressing the role of social determinants (Norheim & Asada, 2009). This necessitates addressing social determinants of health to control and eliminate NTDs, which are a key deterrent in the attainment of global health equity. The need to integrate medical and social interventions becomes significant in this regard. While there is a consensus and acceptance of the medical interventions for NTD control and prevention, there is little consensus and acknowledgement regarding the need for a practice-based discipline to address the question of community engagement for successful NTD interventions. Positioning social work as an essential practice that can address the community participation and adherence requirements of the NTD control and prevention programme requires a set of unique efforts from social work academics and practitioners. Given the disproportionate impact of NTDs on marginalised populations, social work interventions can successfully engage in community organisation that addresses the social determinants that affect the health outcomes of these populations. However, positing NTD social work as an essential practice involves raising awareness, building capacity, advocating for policy changes and fostering collaboration across sectors. This section deals with some of the essential steps to advocate for NTD social work.

(a) *Training and Education*: The first and foremost task in establishing NTD social work is the incorporation of NTD social work into the curriculum. While the present social work education equips the students with medical social work practices and community social work practices, NTDs require social work models that integrate the strengths of both medical and community social work. In addition, NTD social work need not necessarily be a priority in most parts of the world, particularly developed nations. In such a scenario, taking the indigenous context is essential to accommodate NTD social work into the curriculum of developing countries that are endemic to NTDs. As discussed in Chap. 3, there should be efforts to induct modules on social determinants of health, health equity and health promotion with special emphasis on NTDs into the social work curriculum of endemic countries. This can be achieved only through concerted efforts from social work academics and associations to prioritise NTD social work as an essential academic component in endemic countries. Continuing education programmes like Open Online Courses offered by academic bodies can be an effective medium to build NTD social work capacity in developing countries.

(b) *Standardising Practices*: As discussed earlier, medical and community social work practices are compartmentalised in most settings. In order to address NTDs, theories and applications of both medical and community social work practice must be integrated. However, there is no standard set of practices that are laid down when it comes to NTDs in the current state. There needs to be an exploration of the current social work practice models associated with NTDs, and they should be codified into a set of standard practices with theoretical inputs from medical and community social work practices. Chapter 3 of this book lays down a set of basic standards and ground rules regarding NTD social work practice. The key is to evaluate the present models from the field and build upon them in line with social work theories. Collaboration and knowledge-sharing among social work researchers, practitioners and educators are essential in advancing standardisation efforts. Through these concerted efforts, the social work discipline can position itself as a well-codified social science discipline that effectively addresses the social determinants of health in NTDs by projecting it as an essential player in NTD control and elimination efforts.

(c) *Research and Evidence Generation*: As discussed in previous sections, there is limited evidence in the literature regarding the efficacy of social work interventions in the control and elimination efforts of NTDs, despite the active work of social workers in this regard. In order to project the role and efficacy of social work interventions in NTD control and prevention, evidence needs to be generated through research. Social workers are actively involved in interventions that directly target NTD elimination and also in projects that seek to improve social conditions like poverty and access to clean water and sanitation, which have an immense role in the control and elimination of NTDs. The specific impact of these interventions on NTD control and elimination has not been extensively researched or documented. Initiating social work research in order to record the impact of these interventions can serve as the foundation for establishing evidence for the efficacy of NTD social work. Research in this domain shall address multiple domains of NTD social work, including the effectiveness of social work interventions in improving social determinants of health, effective integration of NTD social work with other health interventions like medical interventions and vector control measures, long-term sustainability of social work interventions and cost-effectiveness. Once NTD social work can be established with research-based evidence to be efficacious, sustainable and cost-effective and complement other healthcare interventions, the advocacy for NTD social work will be more effective.

(d) *Advocacy on a Global Stage*: Advocating for NTD social work and the inclusion of social workers in NTD prevention programmes are crucial for addressing the multidimensional challenges associated with these diseases. The first and foremost step in the advocacy involves highlighting the role of social determinants in NTD prevention programs and emphasising how integrating social workers into interventions can address these underlying social determinants more effectively. The second step is to demonstrate the value of social work expertise in NTD control and prevention by advocating for the unique expertise and skill set that social workers bring to NTD prevention efforts. Social workers are trained to understand the complex interplay between individual, social and environmental factors that influence health outcomes. They can provide psychosocial support, community engagement, advocacy and capacity-building services that complement medical interventions in NTD prevention programmes. Thirdly, advocate for integrating evidence-based social work interventions like community-based health education, behaviour change communication, psychosocial support and community mobilisation into NTD prevention programmes. Showcasing the evidence base for social work interventions can strengthen the case for the inclusion of NTD social work in prevention programs. The inclusion of social work indicators in monitoring and evaluation frameworks for NTD prevention programmes can be a good step in this regard. Finally, advocating for the involvement of social workers in policy development and decision-making processes related to NTD prevention should also be done to ensure that NTD social work is acknowledged in policy documents and programme protocols.

(e) *Developing Social Work Infrastructure*: One of the fundamental reasons for the poor recognition of social work practices in the field of NTDs is the lack of social work infrastructure in most developing nations where NTDs are prevalent. In order to argue the case for NTD social work, the professional body in the country should be well established and structured to advocate the subject matter in relevant platforms. A well-developed social work infrastructure ensures that social workers can advocate for increased funding and resources to support the integration of social workers into NTD prevention programs. Likewise, positioning social work as an essential profession in controlling and preventing NTDs would require resources and organised efforts, which can be challenging without a developed social work infrastructure. While the development of such an infrastructure seems challenging, it is essential to ensure the recognition of social work, not just in the realm of NTDs but in general.

(f) *Partnership with NTD Organisations*: Partnering with global players in NTD control and prevention can help social work garner recognition as an essential profession. This can be beneficial to the social work profession in two ways, viz. partnerships with global bodies like the WHO can help disseminate the relevance of social work for addressing social determinants of health in NTD control and prevention and also partnerships with funding agencies can help in advocating for the inclusion of social workers in the multi-disciplinary teams that work on NTDs. Such partnerships can help address the funding challenges many countries face that lead to limited inclusion of social workers in NTD programmes. Building coalitions can effectively promote the inclusion of social workers in NTD prevention programs at the global level.

In order to integrate NTD social work into the framework of NTD programmes, a multifaceted approach involving consorted efforts from academics, practitioners and educators is necessary. From the social work education perspective, incorporating NTD-focused modules into social work education and standardising practices to effectively blend medical and community social work theories are required. From a social work research perspective, efforts must be intensified to provide evidence for the efficacy and impact of social work interventions in combating NTDs. From a social work practitioner perspective, the development of social work infrastructure in endemic regions is crucial for promoting the profession's recognition and ensuring adequate support for practitioners. By collectively addressing these aspects, NTD social work can be positioned as an essential discipline in tackling neglected tropical diseases and advancing health equity worldwide.

4.4 Theoretical Trajectories for Advancing NTD Social Work Practice

The previous sections delved into the challenges and outlined potential pathways for advancing NTD social work. However, in order to advance NTD social work, the first and foremost task is to lay down a theoretical platform. This section delves into the theoretical underpinnings that could inform NTD social work practice. Since NTD social work is not well established as a specialised social work practice globally and also since it is not well recorded in social work literature, there is no consensus regarding the guiding theories. However, drawing from the background of NTDs and the underlying principles of social work, broader social work theories can be adapted for NTD social work practice. This theoretical background for NTD social work shall be perceived as a framework that shall help practitioners address the 'socially constructed' nature of NTDs and the impact of social determinants on the health of individuals. Hence, an overarching rights-based approach is suggested as the cross-cutting theory upon which other theories are superimposed (Fig. 4.1). A potential theoretical ground for NTD social work is depicted in Fig. 4.1 and discussed in this section. While these theories are well established and predominantly applied in social work practice in general, this section aims to explain their relevance and importance in NTD social work practice. However, these theories are not to be considered arbitrarily as the sole theoretical ground but should be considered as a foundation upon which NTD social work can be built in an eclectic manner.

4.4.1 Rights-Based Approach for NTD Social Work

A rights-based approach to social work focuses on transforming societies through efforts to establish care systems based on respect and dignity of all individuals at all times (Gabel, 2023). The approach ensures that the principles of dignity, non-discrimination, participation, transparency and accountability are observed (McPherson, 2020) and founded on the premise that the participation of the impacted sections of society is essential in creating systems that ensure economic, social and environmental justice (Gabel, 2023). One of the fundamental features demarcating NTDs from other public health issues is their intricate entanglement with human rights. It is well established that most NTDs are prevalent in regions marked by

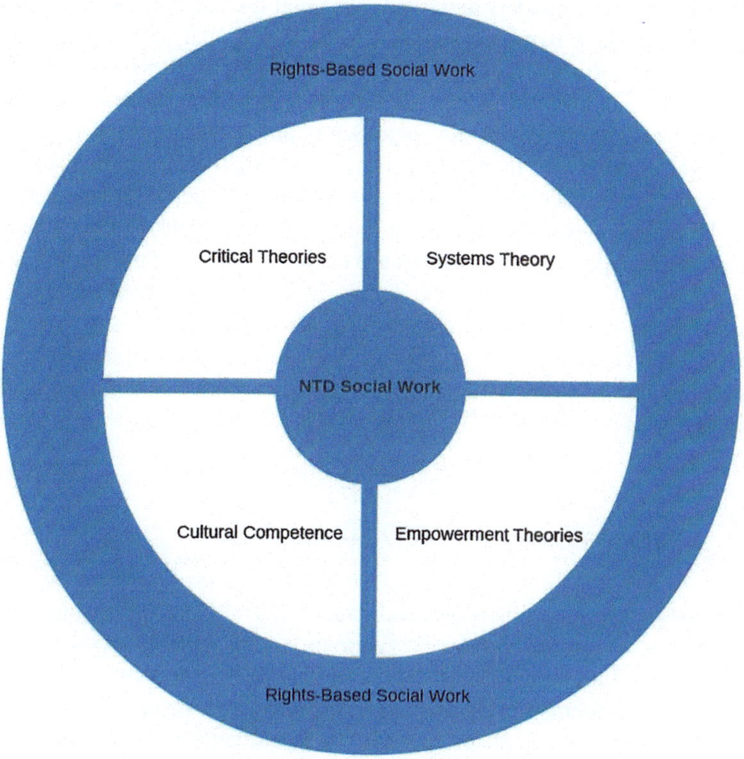

Fig. 4.1 Theoretical grounds for advancing NTD social work

poverty and poor resources, including water and sanitation facilities. This makes NTDs a subject matter of human rights, encompassing the right to life and the right to health. This nexus between NTDs and human rights throws light on the intersectionality of health and social justice for marginalised people. The prevalence of NTDs is a pointer to the shortcomings of governance, public health system and resource allocation, among others. Addressing NTDs from a human-rights perspective helps social workers understand the problem holistically and address the root causes rather than work as an ancillary service to medical interventions. Hence, adopting a rights-based approach as the foundational theoretical ground can help in centring NTD social work on human rights principles to ensure health equity.

A human rights-based approach empowers people to assert their rights and enhances the capacity of institutions to fulfil their obligations under human rights law by practising the principles of participation, accountability, non-discrimination and equality, empowerment and legality, represented by the acronym PANEL (Scottish Human Rights Commission, n.d.). It ensures (a) people can participate in the decision-making processes that affect their rights, (b) constant monitoring and course correction in cases where people's rights are affected, (c) people are treated equally, with those facing severe rights violations treated as a priority, (d) empowering people to understand their rights and take part in developing policies that can impact their lives and (e) adherence to regional and international laws (Scottish Human Rights Commission, n.d.). By adopting this framework, NTD social workers can posit NTDs as a human rights issue first rather than a mere biological disease. The benefit of this approach is that it ensures that the problem of NTDs is addressed from a human rights angle, thereby forcing changes in the structural deficits that induce the vicious cycle of adverse social determinants and ill health. The social work profession, by the very nature of its founding principles, emphasises that human needs are not just a choice but are fundamentally imperative to justice, thereby placing human rights at the centre of its professional practice (United Nations Centre for Human Rights, 1994). This outlook is essential and foundational in NTD social work, which deals with a complex interplay of human needs and health inequity. With rights-based social work as the foundation, other theories serve as pointers for NTD social workers.

4.4.2 Systems Theory for NTD Social Work

Systems theory is a theoretical approach emerging from and applicable to multiple social sciences disciplines and involves studying social phenomena by analysing the interactions and interdependencies between various components within a system (Forder, 1976). Systems theory perceives social systems to be dynamic and intertwined, composed of elements that are constantly influencing each other and thereby shaping the system of which they are part. The application of systems theory in social work practice can help address the question of social change from the lens of power and control (Leighninger, 1977). By emphasising the concept of holism, systems theory argues that a social system is composed of components that are constantly interacting and interdependent on each other, shaping a system that is more than the sum of individual parts (Von Bertalanffy, 1972). Often perceived as an alternative to the medical model of social work, systems theory focuses on the balance between the organism and the individual, acting as a common ground (Leighninger, 1977). In the previous sections, the importance of integrating medical and community social work models for a successful NTD social work model was explained, and systems theory can serve as a theoretical common ground in this aspect.

Individual behaviour, often in resource-limited settings, leads to vulnerability to NTDs, and individual hygiene practices happen in the context of a community. Water, sanitation and hygiene (WASH) is a critical component in the prevention of many NTDs (Salou Bachirou et al., 2023) and promoting WASH essentially involves two components. The first is the development of infrastructure to ensure universal access to water and sanitation, and the second is to induce behavioural change to promote hygiene practices. NTD social work necessarily focuses on both these aspects. By addressing the question of power and control from a systems perspective, NTD social workers can address the structural deficits that restrict social change in this regard. In the domain of behavioural change, systems theory can help social workers address how multiple disadvantages within the system intersect to affect communities. Systems theory can help address how larger components like socio-cultural aspects intersect with individual components to induce vulnerability to NTDs. Thus, systems theory could offer a common ground for community and medical social work models effectively addressing the individual and larger contexts of NTDs.

4.4.3 Critical Theories for NTD Social Work

Critical theory denotes a set of theories that analyse and transform society through an integration of normative perspectives with empirically grounded examinations of the conflicts, contradictions and trends within the society (Celikates & Flynn, 2023). Drawing from the works of Marx, Hegel and Kant, among others, critical theories, in general, aim to critically examine and reveal the dynamics of power and control in which humanity is entrenched (Ryoo & McLaren, 2010). Critical social work refers to the application of critical theories to challenge oppression and bring about social change by empowering communities (Fook, 2003). It seeks to address not only the individual needs of clients but also the broader social, economic, and political factors that contribute to inequality and marginalisation. Some of the guiding principles of critical social work include (a) social justice, (b) empowerment, (c) intersectionality, (d) activism and advocacy and (e) participatory approach. Multiple critical theories are employed in social work, and intersectionality theory is often positioned as an ideal critical ground to address economic and social disparities originating from oppression and privilege (Murphy-Erby et al., 2009). Intersectionality theory, in summary, examines how various social identities, such as race, gender, class and sexuality, intersect and interact to shape individuals' experiences of privilege and oppression (Crenshaw, 2013). The theory is extensively being used in research and practice related to health equity (Lundberg, 2020), making it a good theoretical platform for NTD social work. However, intersectionality theory is not the critical social work approach, and NTD social workers often have to be eclectic when choosing the theoretical grounds for critical social work.

Application of critical theories in NTD social work involves addressing the oppression and privilege leading to poor health outcomes in communities where NTDs are endemic. NTDs are not just diseases but are often the outcome of oppressive structures that limit certain sections of society from attaining a dignified life. NTDs often involve a combination of disproportionate resource allocation, spatial injustice, oppressive social structures and complicit political economy. Hence, addressing NTDs essentially involves addressing these oppressive structures as well. Critical social work practice, with its emphasis on social action and advocacy, offers a comprehensive approach to address these factors. Hence, critical theories offer an important theoretical ground for NTD social work. The application of critical theories in NTD social work involves recognising NTDs as manifestations of broader social injustices and working towards transformative change that addresses the underlying structural determinants of health. By adopting a critical lens, social workers can play a crucial role in advocating for the rights and dignity of communities affected by NTDs and fostering conditions that enable all individuals to lead healthy and fulfilling lives.

4.4.4 Cultural Competence Theory for NTD Social Work

Cultural competence refers to the framework used in fields like social work, psychology and education to address cultural diversity effectively. Cultural competence demands individuals and systems to engage with people from diverse backgrounds in a respectful and effective manner (Gallegos et al., 2008). It emphasises the importance of individuals and organisations being able to interact with people from diverse backgrounds effectively. The National Association of Social Workers (2015, p. 13) defines cultural competence as 'the process by which individuals and systems respond respectfully and effectively to people of all cultures, languages, classes, races, ethnic backgrounds, religions, spiritual traditions, immigration status, and other diversity factors in a manner that recognises, affirms, and values the worth of individuals, families, and communities and protects and preserves the dignity of each'. Cultural competence demands that practitioners be aware of their own worldview and any biases or assumptions originating from it and understand the worldviews of people from diverse backgrounds non-judgementally with a sense of cultural humility (National Association of Social Workers, 2015). Social work emphasises cultural competence, and social workers are trained to address cultural diversity in their practice.

In the context of NTDs, it could be seen that control and prevention efforts need to address the cultural components of the targeted population to deliver interventions effectively. Gaining community acceptability is one of the key factors in the successful implementation of preventive strategies like MDA, and one of the major reasons for poor adherence is the lack of cultural understanding (Niles et al., 2021; Abdul Halim et al., 2022). NTD social work, with its emphasis on cultural competence, can address the cultural component of NTDs effectively, thereby strengthening control and elimination measures. With the regional diversities within countries being extensive in many Asian and African nations that are endemic to NTDs, it is essential that control and elimination efforts deliver interventions in a tailor-made manner that addresses the cultural components of the communities under consideration. NTD social work can be pivotal in bringing this cultural competence to NTD control and prevention efforts and improving the efficacy of programmes like MDA.

4.4.5 *Empowerment Theories for NTD Social Work*

Empowerment involves enabling individuals or communities to access resources in order to make choices that can enhance their control over their lives. Empowerment theories place individual well-being in the context of the political and social environment, i.e. the theory postulates that transformations in the social and political environment are essential in attaining individual well-being (Perkins & Zimmerman, 1995). Empowerment can be both a process and an outcome. The actions taken or activities done themselves can be empowering, and the outcome of such processes can lead to a state of empowerment (Zimmerman, 2000). The process of empowerment entails identifying power blocks that contribute to the issues, along with devising and executing particular strategies to address them (Solomon, 1976). The power blocks could be either 'direct', involving structures that directly prevent a community from attaining certain goals for their betterment, or 'indirect', involving internalised oppression of groups that have a history of marginalisation (Solomon, 1976; Rozario, 1997). Empowerment approaches entail collective action against oppressive social structures, thereby enabling people to gain greater control over their lives (Rozario, 1997)

Empowerment theories are applied in social work practice to address individual challenges like internalised psychological distress and also to address community challenges like empowering marginalised communities. With its emphasis on both individual aspects and community aspects, NTD social work can empower endemic communities. Most NTDs are prevalent among communities that are disadvantaged and marginalised over generations. They face both direct and indirect power blocks due to the complex social structures in the endemic countries. Addressing this aspect is key in bringing about structural changes at the community level and behavioural change at the individual level. With its emphasis on empowerment, NTD social work can address this component effectively.

Laying down a theoretical platform is paramount for the progress of NTD social work. While theories described in this section are essential in NTD social work, it is desirable that an eclectic approach integrating these theories be applied for effective practice. Each theoretical framework offers unique insights and tools for understanding and addressing the complex interplay of social, economic and political factors contributing to NTD prevalence and impact. Emphasising human rights principles, acknowledging the systemic nature of health disparities, challenging oppressive structures, promoting cultural humility and empowering individuals and communities are integral aspects of NTD social work practice. By adopting a comprehensive and interdisciplinary approach informed by these theoretical perspectives, social workers can contribute effectively to the control and eradication of NTDs and the promotion of health equity on a global scale.

4.5 Conclusion

This chapter has examined the future directions and theoretical trajectories crucial for the evolution and effectiveness of NTD social work. While factors like limited evidence regarding the effectiveness of NTD social work, poor social work infrastructure in most countries affected with NTDs and dominance of medical models pose significant challenges in establishing NTD social work as core practice, the unique skillset of social work can be projected by increased evidence generation through research efforts and advocating for the inclusion of social workers in the public health teams. For effective NTD social work practice, theoretical frameworks such as the rights-based approach, systems theory, critical theories, cultural competence theory and empowerment theories should be put to use for understanding and addressing the multifaceted nature of NTDs and their impact on individuals and communities. By adopting an eclectic approach that integrates these theories, social workers can navigate the intricate dynamics of NTDs, advocate for social justice, challenge oppressive structures and empower individuals and communities towards better health outcomes.

References

Abdul Halim, A. F. N., Ahmad, D., Miaw Yn, J. L., Masdor, N. A., Ramly, N., Othman, R., et al. (2022). Factors associated with the acceptability of mass drug administration for filariasis: A systematic review. *International Journal of Environmental Research and Public Health, 19*(19), 12971.

Allotey, P., Reidpath, D. D., & Pokhrel, S. (2010). Social sciences research in neglected tropical diseases 1: The ongoing neglect in the neglected tropical diseases. *Health Research Policy and Systems, 8*(32), 1–8. https://doi.org/10.1186/1478-4505-8-32

Baikady, R., Cheng, S. L., & Channaveer, R. M. (2020). Eight decades of existence and search for an identity: Educators perspectives on social work education in contemporary India. *Social Work Education, 40*(8), 994–1009. https://doi.org/10.1080/02615479.2020.1773780

Blom, B. R. (2004). Specialization in social work practice: Effects on interventions in the personal social services. *Journal of Social Work, 4*(1), 25–46.

Celikates, R., & Flynn, J. (2023). Critical theory (Frankfurt School). In E. N. Zalta & U. Nodelman (Eds.), *The Stanford encyclopedia of philosophy*. Retrieved from https://plato.stanford.edu/entries/critical-theory/

Chitereka, C. (2009). Social work in a developing continent: The case of Africa. *Advances in Social Work, 10*(2), 144–156.

Crenshaw, K. (2013). Demarginalizing the intersection of race and sex: A black feminist critique of antidiscrimination doctrine, feminist theory and antiracist politics. In *Feminist legal theories* (pp. 23–51). Routledge.

Fleming, C., Young, S., Else, J., Hammond, L., & McLaren, H. (2023). A yarn among social workers: Knowing, being, and doing social work learning, expertise, and practice. *Australian Social Work, 76*(3), 330–342.

Fook, J. (2003). Critical social work: The current issues. *Qualitative Social Work, 2*(2), 123–130.

Forder, A. (1976). Social work and system theory. *The British Journal of Social Work, 6*(1), 23–42.

Gabel, S. G. (2023). *A human rights-based approach to justice in social work practice*. Oxford University Press.

Gallegos, J. S., Tindall, C., & Gallegos, S. A. (2008). The need for advancement in the conceptualization of cultural competence. *Advances in Social Work, 9*(1), 51–62.

Ioakimidis, V., & Sookraj, D. (2021). Global standards for social work education and training. *International Social Work, 64*(2), 161–174.

Leighninger, R. D. (1977). Systems theory and social work: A reexamination. *Journal of Education for Social Work, 13*(3), 44–49.

Lundberg, O. (2020). Next steps in the development of the social determinants of health approach: The need for a new narrative. *Scandinavian Journal of Public Health, 48*(5), 473–479. https://doi.org/10.1177/1403494819894789

Mathew, A. (2020, November 9). Modi government circulates draft Bill to regulate autonomy in social work practice, education. *National Herald.* Retrieved from https://www.nationalheraldindia.com/india/modi-government-circulates-draft-bill-to-regulate-autonomy-in-social-work-practice-education. Accessed 5 June 2024.

McPherson, J. (2020). Now is the time for a rights-based approach to social work practice. *Journal of Human Rights and Social Work, 5*, 61–63.

Mitchell, E., Kelly-Hanku, A., Krentel, A., Romani, L., Robinson, L. J., Vaz Nery, S., Kaldor, J., Steer, A. C., & Bell, S. (2022). Community perceptions and acceptability of mass drug administration for the control of neglected tropical diseases in Asia-Pacific countries: A systematic scoping review of qualitative research. *PLoS Neglected Tropical Diseases, 16*(3), e0010215. https://doi.org/10.1371/journal.pntd.0010215

Molyneux, D. H., Asamoa-Bah, A., Fenwick, A., Savioli, L., & Hotez, P. (2021). The history of the neglected tropical disease movement. *Transactions of the Royal Society of Tropical Medicine and Hygiene, 115*(2), 169–175.

Murphy-Erby, Y., Hunt, V., Zajicek, A., Norris, A., & Hamilton, L. (2009). *Incorporating intersectionality in social work practice, research, policy, and education.* NASW Press.

National Association of Social Workers. (2015). *Standards and indicators for cultural competence in social work practice.* NASW Press.

Nikku, B. R., & Pulla, V. (2014). Global agenda for social work and social development: Voices of the social work educators from Asia. *International Social Work, 57*(4), 373–385.

Niles, R. A., Thickstun, C. R., Cox, H., Dilliott, D., Burgert-Brucker, C. R., Harding-Esch, E. M., et al. (2021). Assessing factors influencing communities' acceptability of mass drug administration for the elimination of lymphatic filariasis in Guyana. *PLoS Neglected Tropical Diseases, 15*(9), e0009596.

Norheim, O. F., & Asada, Y. (2009). The ideal of equal health revisited: Definitions and measures of inequity in health should be better integrated with theories of distributive justice. *International Journal for Equity in Health, 8*(1), 1–9.

Perkins, D. D., & Zimmerman, M. A. (1995). Empowerment theory, research, and application. *American Journal of Community Psychology, 23*, 569–579.

Rozario, S. (1997). Development and rural women in South Asia: The limits of empowerment and conscientization. *Bulletin of Concerned Asian Scholars, 29*(4), 45–53.

Ruth, B. J., & Marshall, J. W. (2017). A history of social work in public health. *American Journal of Public Health, 107*(S3), S236–S242.

Ryoo, J. J., & McLaren, P. (2010). Critical theory. In P. Peterson, E. Baker, & B. McGaw (Eds.), *International encyclopedia of education* (pp. 348–353). Elsevier. https://doi.org/10.1016/B978-0-08-044894-7.01388-9

Salou Bachirou, Z., Mignanwande, Z. F., Bokossa, H., Degnonvi, H., Djossou, P., Hondjrebo, F., et al. (2023). WASH and NTDs: Outcomes and lessons learned from the implementation of a formative research study in NTD skin co-endemic communities in Benin. *Frontiers in Medicine, 10*, 1022314.

Scottish Human Rights Commission. (n.d.). *A human rights based approach: An introduction.* Retrieved from https://www.scottishhumanrights.com/media/1409/shrc_hrba_leaflet.pdf

Solomon, B. B. (1976). *Black empowerment: Social work in oppressed communities.* Columbia University Press.

Taylor, M., Thomas, R., Oliver, S., & Garner, P. (2022). Community views on mass drug administration for filariasis: A qualitative evidence synthesis. *The Cochrane Database of Systematic Reviews, 2*(2), CD013638. https://doi.org/10.1002/14651858.CD013638.pub2

United Nations Centre for Human Rights (Ed.). (1994). *Human rights and social work: A manual for schools of social work and the social work profession*. United Nations.

Von Bertalanffy, L. (1972). The history and status of general systems theory. *Academy of Management Journal, 15*(4), 407–426.

Zimmerman, M. A. (2000). Empowerment theory. In J. Rappaport & E. Seidman (Eds.), *Handbook of community psychology* (pp. 43–63). Springer US. https://doi.org/10.1007/978-1-4615-4193-6_2

Chapter 5
Conclusion

The critical intersection of medical and social dimensions in the case of neglected tropical diseases (NTDs) affect the world's poorest populations, where inadequate sanitation, limited healthcare facilities and financial constraints exacerbate their impact (Hotez, 2021). NTDs exert a significant strain on the healthcare system, as most affected countries are low- or middle-income countries with limited healthcare infrastructure. The impact of NTDs on the affected individuals and communities is also significant, as NTDs often leads to a vicious cycle of poverty and poor health outcomes (Hotez et al., 2014). The social dimensions, including poverty, cultural practices and social identity, significantly influence disease dynamics and outcomes, as evidenced by the situation in India (Acharya et al., 2017). In order to address this 'socially constructed' aspect of NTDs, integrating social work into NTD interventions can help. Social workers bring unique strengths in understanding socio-cultural dynamics, fostering community engagement and advocating for policy changes. These contributions can effectively address the complex web of factors affecting NTD prevalence and outcomes.

However, social work is not often recognised as pertinent profession in NTD interventions in most of the affected countries due to multiple factors including lack of recognition of the profession in general, a dearth of literature and research on the impact of NTD social work, among other factors (Nikku & Pulla, 2014; Chitereka, 2009). Such limitations exist in almost all the Asian and African nations where NTDs are prevalent. The integration of social work into NTD interventions could provide much-needed support for communities grappling with these diseases, yet the profession remains underutilised and undervalued. To effectively combat NTDs, a paradigm shift is needed that recognises the critical role of social work in public health. By integrating social workers into NTD intervention strategies, more holistic and sustainable solutions can be devised. Social workers can bridge the gap between medical and social dimensions of health, ensuring that interventions are culturally

© The Author(s), under exclusive license to Springer Nature Switzerland AG 2024

M. Jabir, A. C. Choolayil, *Social Work with Populations Vulnerable to Neglected Tropical Diseases*, SpringerBriefs in Social Work,
https://doi.org/10.1007/978-3-031-68997-0_5

sensitive and community driven. This approach can both addresses the immediate health needs of affected populations and help tackle the root causes of disease transmission and persistence. Integrating social work interventions into NTD programmes also aligns with the public health strategy of emphasising the role of social determinants in shaping health outcomes.

To establish NTD social work as an essential practice, efforts must be directed towards training and education, standardising practices, research and evidence generation, advocacy on a global stage, developing social work infrastructure and fostering partnerships with NTD organisations. These endeavours are indispensable for embedding NTD social work into the framework of NTD programmes and ensuring its recognition and efficacy in addressing the complex social determinants of health underlying NTD prevalence. Social workers can navigate the intricate dynamics of NTDs, advocate for social justice, challenge oppressive structures and empower individuals and communities towards better health outcomes. The establishment and advancement of NTD social work necessitate collaborative efforts from academics, practitioners, educators and policymakers. By collectively addressing the outlined future directions and drawing from theoretical trajectories, NTD social work can emerge as a formidable force in the global fight against neglected tropical diseases, contributing significantly to the promotion of health equity and social justice worldwide.

References

Acharya, A. S., Kaur, R., & Goel, A. D. (2017). Neglected tropical diseases—Challenges and opportunities in India. *Indian Journal of Medical Specialities, 8*(3), 102–108.

Chitereka, C. (2009). Social work in a developing continent: The case of Africa. *Advances in Social Work, 10*(2), 144–156.

Hotez, P. J. (2021). *Forgotten people, forgotten diseases: The neglected tropical diseases and their impact on global health and development.* Wiley.

Hotez, P. J., Alvarado, M., Basáñez, M. G., Bolliger, I., Bourne, R., Boussinesq, M., et al. (2014). The global burden of disease study 2010: Interpretation and implications for the neglected tropical diseases. *PLoS Neglected Tropical Diseases, 8*(7), e2865.

Nikku, B. R., & Pulla, V. (2014). Global agenda for social work and social development: Voices of the social work educators from Asia. *International Social Work, 57*(4), 373–385.

Glossary

Behavioural Determinants Actions or habits that influence health outcomes, such as lifestyle choices, hygiene practices and treatment-seeking behaviours.

Case Management Providing medical care, treatment and support services to individuals with specific health needs, coordinating various aspects of their care.

Capacity Building Developing skills, knowledge and abilities in organisations or communities to improve health outcomes.

Community Engagement The process of working in collaboration with community groups to address issues affecting their well-being.

Cultural Competence The ability to understand, communicate with and effectively interact with people across different cultures, respecting their beliefs, practices and customs.

DALYs (Disability Adjusted Life Years) A measure disease burden, calculated as the number of years lost due to ill health, disability or early death.

Disease Surveillance The continuous, systematic collection, analysis and interpretation of health-related data.

Epidemiology The study of the distribution and determinants of health-related states and events in populations.

Ethical Standards Guidelines for proper conduct in research and practice, ensuring respect, fairness and integrity.

Health Advocacy Activities that seek to influence health policy, planning and service delivery.

Health Education Education that promotes awareness, knowledge and skills related to health and wellness.

Health Equity The principle of providing fair opportunities for health for everyone and eliminating disparities in health outcomes.

Health Inequity Avoidable differences in health between different groups of people, often caused by social, economic and environmental conditions.

© The Editor(s) (if applicable) and The Author(s), under exclusive license to Springer Nature Switzerland AG 2024

M. Jabir, A. C. Choolayil, *Social Work with Populations Vulnerable to Neglected Tropical Diseases*, SpringerBriefs in Social Work,
https://doi.org/10.1007/978-3-031-68997-0

Health Policy Decisions, plans and actions undertaken to achieve specific health-care goals within a society.

Intersectoral Collaboration Cooperation among different sectors (e.g., health, education environment) to address health issues.

Lymphatic Filariasis A parasitic disease transmitted by mosquitoes, resulting in severe swelling in the limbs and genitals.

Mass Drug Administration (MDA) The administration of drugs to entire populations in a geographical area to control and eliminate disease.

Neglected Tropical Diseases (NTDs) A group of infections prevalent in tropical and subtropical regions, resulting in significant health burdens.

One Health An approach that recognises that the health of humans, animals and ecosystems are interconnected.

Public Health The science of preventing disease, prolonging life and promoting health through organised efforts.

Public-Private Partnerships (PPP) Collaborative projects between government and private sector entities to improve public health outcomes.

Sanitation Measures designed to protect public health by maintaining sanitation and preventing human contact with hazardous waste.

Social Determinants of Health Conditions in which people are born, grow, live, work and/or age, which impact their health.

Stigma The process of devaluation of individuals based on certain attributes or characteristics they possess, resulting in discrimination.

Sustainable Development Goals (SDGs) A set of 17 goals set by the United Nations to address global challenges, including health.

Urbanisation The process of population concentration in urban areas, often accompanied by infrastructure development and socio-economic changes.

Vector Control Methods to control or eliminate disease vectors, such as insects, to prevent disease transmission.

Vector-Borne Diseases Diseases transmitted to humans and other animals by blood-feeding arthropods, such as mosquitoes, ticks and fleas.

Visceral Leishmaniasis (VL) A vector-borne disease caused by parasites and transmitted by sandfly bites.

Zoonotic Diseases A set of diseases that can be transmitted from animals to humans.

Index

© The Editor(s) (if applicable) and The Author(s), under exclusive license to Springer Nature Switzerland AG 2024
M. Jabir, A. C. Choolayil, *Social Work with Populations Vulnerable to Neglected Tropical Diseases*, SpringerBriefs in Social Work,
https://doi.org/10.1007/978-3-031-68997-0

SPRINGER NATURE

GPSR Compliance

The European Union's (EU) General Product Safety Regulation (GPSR) is a set of rules that requires consumer products to be safe and our obligations to ensure this.

If you have any concerns about our products, you can contact us on ProductSafety@springernature.com

In case Publisher is established outside the EU, the EU authorized representative is:

Springer Nature Customer Service Center GmbH
Europaplatz 3
69115 Heidelberg, Germany

The manufacturer's authorised representative in the EU is Springer Nature Customer Service Centre GmbH, Europaplatz 3, 69115 Heidelberg, Germany. If you have any concerns regarding our products, please contact ProductSafety@springernature.com

Printed and bound by CPI Group (UK) Ltd, Croydon, CR0 4YY
01/10/2026
02225985-0001